Pocketbook of

Ayurvedic Medicine Reckoner

For Ayurvedic Practitioners and Professionals

Pocketbook of
Ayurvedic Medicine Reckoner

For Ayurvedic Practitioners and Professionals

Pravesh Kumar Mukeriya
BAMS MD (Ayu) Panchakarma
Associate Professor
PG Department of Panchakarma
Uttarakhand Ayurved University
Rishikul Campus, Haridwar, Uttarakhand, India

JAYPEE

JAYPEE BROTHERS MEDICAL PUBLISHERS
The Health Sciences Publisher
New Delhi | London

Jaypee Brothers Medical Publishers (P) Ltd

Headquarters
EMCA House
23/23-B, Ansari Road, Daryaganj
New Delhi 110 002, India
Landline: +91-11-23272143, +91-11-23272703
+91-11-23282021, +91-11-23245672
E-mail: jaypee@jaypeebrothers.com

Corporate Office
4838/24, Ansari Road, Daryaganj
New Delhi 110 002, India
Phone: +91-11-43574357
Fax: +91-11-43574314
E-mail: jaypee@jaypeebrothers.com

Overseas Office
J.P. Medical Ltd
83 Victoria Street, London
SW1H 0HW (UK)
Phone: +44 20 3170 8910
E-mail: info@jpmedpub.com

EU GPSR Authorised Representative
Logos Europe, 9 rue Nicolas Poussin
17000, La Rochelle, France
Phone: +33 (0) 6 67 93 73 78
E-mail: contact@logoseurope.eu

Website: www.jaypeebrothers.com
Website: www.jaypeedigital.com

Inquiries for bulk sales may be solicited at: jaypee@jaypeebrothers.com

Pocketbook of Ayurvedic Medicine Reckoner for Ayurvedic Practitioners and Professionals

First Edition: **2021**

Reprint: **2026**

ISBN 978-93-90595-60-0

Printed at: Samrat Offset Pvt. Ltd.

Dedicated to

My parents

Shri SR Singh and Late Smt Shimla Devi

and

my all the teachers

Preface

Ayurveda is an ancient and rich medical system that has been serving mankind in the treatment of different diseases for thousands of years. In this system of medicine, mainly medicinal plants as well as metals and minerals are used for medicinal purposes after so many detoxification processes to make them safe and effective for internal use of humans.

In the book, different medicinal formulations and preparations used in ayurvedic clinical practice, their standard dose and important indications are given. Also, medicines indicated in case of different diseases or clinical conditions have been described in respect of their indications and standard dose.

While doing clinical practice, doctor should have a pithy book in which one can easily get a medicinal reference to a disease and its symptoms. This is the purpose of writing this book so that a doctor can easily get medicinal reference in the context of a disease and its specifics including symptomatic treatment in a very short time.

Pravesh Kumar Mukeriya

Acknowledgments

I feel immense pleasure and satisfaction on this small effort as a result of the infinite grace of God, blessings and inspirational values of my parents, blessings of *Gurus*, guidance of the saintly scholars of Ayurveda and the unmatched support of my family members.

I consider it my absolute duty to express my gratitude to all the teachers, doctors and scholars of Ayurveda for invaluable support and guidance in this regard.

I am very grateful to Shri Jitendar P Vij (Group Chairman), Mr Ankit Vij (Managing Director), Mr MS Mani (Group President), Dr Madhu Choudhary (Publishing Head-Education), Ms Pooja Bhandari (Production Head), Ms Sunita Katla (Executive Assistant to Group Chairman and Publishing Manager), Ms Samina Khan (Executive Assistant to Publishing Head-Education), Mr Rajesh Sharma (Production Coordinator), Ms Seema Dogra (Cover Visualizer), Mr Vakil Khan (Proofreader), Mr Ajeet Rathor (Typesetter), and their team members of M/s Jaypee Brothers Medical Publishers (P) Ltd, New Delhi, India, who gave me this opportunity to present my efforts in the form of a pocketbook.

Contents

1 Aushadha Kalpa

Bhasma and Pishti

Abhraka Bhasma

Dose: 1–2 *ratti* (125–250 mg) bid with a suitable *anupana* according to the *roga*.

Indications: *Rajayakshma, kaphakshaya, kasa, urah-kshata, dhatukshaya, svasa, prameha somaroga, pandu, daha, jirnajvara, sangrahni, gulma, agnimandya, paittika vyadhis, hridaya* and *mansika vikara*.

Akika Bhasma and Pishti

Dose: 1–3 *ratti* (125–375 mg) bid with *madhu, makkhana* or according to the *roga*.

Indications: *Hridya-daurbalya, daha, netraroga, raktapitta, mastishka* and *paittika vikara*.

Note: *Pishti* is more efficacious than *bhasma*.

Kapardika Bhasma

Dose: 2–4 *ratti* (250–500 mg) bid with *nimbu* or *tambula svarasa*.

Indications: *Parinamashula, annadravashula, sangrahni, amlapitta, rasakshya, trishna, gulma, karnasrava, udara-vata, mandagni* and *paittika vikara.*

Trinakantamani or Keharva Bhasma and Pishti

Dose: 2–4 *ratti* (250–500 mg) bid–tds with *madhu* or *makkhana.*

Indications: *Raktapitta, paittika vikara, hridaya-daurbalya, chhardi, pravahika, arsha, chakkara, daha, trishnadhikya, atisveda, pittajanya updrava* and *krimijanya shirahshula.*

Kasisa Bhasma

Dose: 1–3 *ratti* (125–375 mg) bid with *madhu.*

Indications: *Pandu, kshaya, kustha, yakrita-pliha vriddhi, ama vikara, udara roga, vrana* and carbuncles.

Kasisa Godanti Bhasma

Dose: 1–3 *ratti* (125–375 mg) bid with *mishri, kshira* or *madhu.*

Indications: *Amajanya nutana jvara, vishamajvara, jirnajvara, pandu, svetapradara, mandagni* and *ama vikara.*

Kansya Bhasma

Dose: 1–2 *ratti* (125–250 mg) bid with *madhu* or *gulkanda.*

Indications: *Krimi, kustha, vata-paittika roga, mandagni, chakshusya, pradara prameha* and *tvag-rukshta.*

Kukkutandatvaka Bhasma

Dose: 2–3 *ratti* (250–375 mg) bid with *madhu.*

Indications: *Prameha, mutraroga, vajikarana, rasayana, shukradosha* and *rajovikara.*

Kharpara Bhasma

Dose: 2–3 *ratti* (250–375 mg) bid with *madhu.*

Indications: *Prameha, netraroga, rajayakshma* and *dhatugata jirnajvara.*

Godanti Hartala Bhasma

Dose: 2–4 *ratti* (250–500 mg) bid with *madhu.*

Indications: *Jvara, pratishyaya, shveta pradara, rakta pradara, shuska kasa, shirah shula, suryavarta* and *ardhavabhedaka.*

Yashada Bhasma

Dose: ½–1 *ratti* (60–125 mg) bid with *madhu, makkhana, malai, mishri* or *roganusara.*

Indications: *Pittanashaka, chakshusya, pandu, pramaha, svasa, granthi, arbuda, daha, pradara, kasa, rajayakshma atisara, sangrahani, dhatukshaya, jirnajvara, kanthamala, apachi* and *abhyantara shotha.*

Jaharmohra Pishti

Dose: 1–2 *ratti* (125–250 mg) bid to qid with *madhu* or *godugdha.*

Indications: *Hridaya* and *mastiska daurbalya, daha, visuchika, atisara, yakrita vikara, ghabrahata, jirnajvara, shosha, shitala* and *raktachapa vriddhi.*

Tamra Bhasma

Dose: ½–1 *ratti* (60–125 mg) bid with *madhu.*

Indications: *Udara roga, prameha, ajirna, vishama jvara, yakrita vikara, parinama shula, hikka, mansarbuda, gulma, kustha, krimi roga, sangrahni, pittashaya roga, asthila* and *jalodara.*

Trivanga Bhasma

Dose: 1–2 *ratti* (125–250 mg) bid with *madhu, makkhana* or *malai.*

Indications: *Prameha, prameha pidika, garbhashaya daurbalya* and *sveta pradara.*

Naga Bhasma

Dose: 1–2 *ratti* (125–250 mg) bid with *madhu, makkhana* or *malai.*

Indications: *Madhumeha, netraroga, gulma, pliha vriddhi, pradara, raktagulma, apachi, gandamala, dhatukshaya, kasa, amavata* and *asthi vikara.*

Pravala Bhasma and Pishti

Dose: *Bhasma* 1–4 *ratti* (125–500 mg), *pishti* 1–6 *ratti* (125–750 mg) bid with *madhu.*

Indications: *Kaphanashaka, pittashamaka, daha, kshaya, raktapitta, kasa, agnimandya, visha, bhutabadha, unmada, pandu, netraroga, hridaya daurbalya, raktachapa vriddhi, paittika vikara, amlapitta, raktapitta jvara* and *rajayakshma.*

Vanga Bhasma

Dose: 1–2 *ratti* (125–250 mg) bid with *madhu.*

Indications: *Mukha daurgandhya, prameha, pandu, gulma, raktapitta, agnimandya, urdhvasvasa, daha, shukrameha, tvagdosha, dhatukshaya, kustha* and *jalodara.*

Vajra Bhasma

Dose: 1 *ratti* of *vajra bhasma* is mixed well with 4 *masha* of *rasasindura* and then used in dose of 1–2 *ratti* (125–250 mg) bid with *madhu.*

Indications: *Arbuda* or *karkatarbuda* and *raktachapa vriddhi.*

Note: *Vaikranta bhasma* may be used as substitute of *vajra bhasma* in the dose of 1–2 *ratti* (125–250 mg).

Mandura Bhasma

Dose: 2–8 *ratti* (250 mg–1 g) bid with *madhu.*

Indications: *Pandu, mandagni, kamala, yakrita* and *pliha vriddhi, arsha* and *rakta vikara.*

Note: *Madhu mandura* is more efficacious than *mandura bhasma* in the dose of 1–6 *ratti* (125–750 mg).

Mayura Chandrika Bhasma

Dose: 2 *ratti* (250 mg) with *madhu.*

Indications: *Hikka, vamana, svasa* and *kasa.*

Mukta Bhasma and Pishti

Dose: 1–2 *ratti* (125–250 mg) with *madhu* or as per the *roga.*

Indications: *Kampavata, drishti daurbalya, paittika vikara anidra, amlapitta, antardaha, rajayakshma, anuloma kshaya, urah kshata, jirnajvara, mutrakricchha* and *garbhopdrava.*

Muktashukti Bhasma and Pishti

Dose: 2–4 *ratti* (250–500 mg) bid with *madhu.*

Indications: *Kshaya, kasa, svasa, jirnajvara, netradaha, hridya roga, paittika vikara, paittika parinama shula, amlapitta, pradara* and *raktaja gulma.*

Rajata Bhasma

Dose: 1 *ratti* (125 mg) bid with *madhu, makkhana* or *mishri.*

Indications: *Daha, vata-pittadhikya, prameha, mastishka daurbalya, pandu, shuska kasa, jvara, udara vata, anidra, unmada, apasmara, snayu daurbalya, hikka* and *garbhasya shodhana.*

Lauha Bhasma

Dose: 1–2 *ratti* (125–250 mg) bid with *madhu.*

Indications: *Pandu, kapha roganashaka, raktapitta, prameha, paittika vikara, sandhigata roga, shotha, dhatu vikara, sangrahni, medovriddhi, mandagni, jirnajvara* and *kamala.*

Shankha Bhasma

Dose: 4–8 *ratti* (500 mg–1 g) bid with *madhu.*

Indications: *Sangrahni, udarashula, yuvana pidika, ajirna, mandagni, amlapitta* and *atisara.*

Sphatika Bhasma

Dose: 2–4 *ratti* (250–500 mg) bid with *madhu.*

Indications: *Sujaka, rakta pradara, kasa, parshvashula, jirna kasa, rajayakshma, phuphaphusa shotha, kukkura kasa, rakta vamana, visha vikara, mutrakricchha, prameha, kustha* and *vrana.*

Shringa Bhasma

Dose: 1–3 *ratti* (125–375 mg) bid with *madhu.*

Indications: *Kasa, svasa, parshvashula, phuphaphusa shotha, svasnika shotha, pratishyaya, jirnajvara, rajayakshma, hridaya-shula* and *urastoya.*

Sangeyashava Bhasma and Pishti

Dose: 2–4 *ratti* (250–500 mg) bid with *madhu* or *mishri.*

Indications: *Hridaya gati vriddhi.*

Sangajarahat Bhasma

Dose: 4–8 *ratti* (500–1000 mg) bid with *makkhana* or *malai.*

Indications: *Raktapitta.*

Hajrulyahuda Bhasma

Dose: 2–4 *ratti* (250–500 mg) bid with *nariyala jala* or *ashmarihara kvatha.*

Indications: *Ashmari, mutrakrichha* and *mutravrodha.*

Svarna Bhasma

Dose: ¼–½ *ratti* (30–60 mg) bid with *madhu, makkhana, mishri* or *malai.*

Indications: *Rasayana, hridya, kshaya, jirnajvara, mastiska daurbalya, daha, paittika roga, kasa* and *svasa.*

Svarnamakshika Bhasma

Dose: 1–2 *ratti* (125–250 mg) bid with *madhu* or *makkhana.*

Indications: *Vrishya,rasayan, yogvahi, pittashamaka, stambhaka, raktaprasadana, pandu, kamala, jirnajvara, pitta vikara, amlapitta, raktapitta, vrana, prameha, pradara, mutrakricchha, visha vikara, kshaya, arsha, udararoga, kustha, krimi* and *madatya.*

Kupipakva Rasayana

Ashtamurti Rasayana

Dose: 1–2 *ratti* (125–250 mg) bid with *adraka svarasa* and *madhu.*

Indications: *Jirna updansha, parivartita jvara, vishama jvara, kshaya, sannipata jvara, sanyasa, bhutonmada, apasmara, mutraghata, kalayakhanja, aptanaka, aptantraka, dhatuskampa* and *phiranga.*

Siddha Makardhvaja

Dose: 1–3 *ratti* (125–375 mg) bid with *tambula patra svarasa, madhu, mishri* or *makkhana.*

Indications: *Jvara, vishama jvara, jirna jvara, jvaratisara, sangrahni, ajirna, vishuchika, rajayakshama, svasa, kasa,* *svarabhanga, unmada, apasmara, vatavyadhi, amavata, hridayaroga, shukrameha* and *murchha.*

Rasasindura

Dose: 1-2 *ratti* (125–250 mg) bid with *madhu.*

Indications: *Jvara, prameha, pradara, unmada, apasmara, svasa, kamala, ajirna, udarashula, murchha, sarvanga shotha, jirna vrana, visphota, amavata, shirah kampa* and *madatya.*

Talasindura

Dose: ½–1 *ratti* (60–125 mg) bid *madhu* or *ardraka svarasa.*

Indications: *Vata vikara, atashaka, vatarakta, vishama jvara, charma roga, urastoya, jalodara* and *rajayakshama.*

Panchasuta Rasa

Dose: ½–1 *ratti* (60–125 mg) bid with *madhu* and *tulsipatra* or *ardraka svarasa.*

Indications: *Svasa, kasa, amajanyashula, vata vyadhi, phuphaphusa avarana shotha, sannipata jvara, balagraha* (*skandagraha, ahiputana,* etc.) and *dhatridosha.*

Malasindura

Dose: ½–1 *ratti* (60–125 mg) bid with *madhu* and *ardraka svarasa.*

Indications: *Vishama jvara, visuchika, phiranga, atashaka, pakshaghata, amavata, dhanurvata, urastoya, yoshapasmara, kaphaja sannipata* and *napunsakta.*

Special precautions: *Pitta pradhanavastha, tivra jvara.*

Tamrasindura

Dose: 1–2 *ratti* (125–250 mg) bid with *madhu* or *tulasipatra svarasa.*

Indications: *Yakrita-pliha roga, udarashula, rajayakshma* of the intestines, *vishuchika, tvakroga, amashaya karkata-sphota, vata-kaphaja mansarbuda, pittashaya shotha, jalodara* of *yakrita-vikara* origin, *kaphaja granthi, visuchika, tivra chhardi, apasmara, bala akshepa* and *rajorodha.*

Shilasindura

Dose: 1–2 *ratti* (125–250 mg) bid with *madhu.*

Indications: *Kustha, tvagroga, kasa, svasa, sthaulya, kanthamala, apachi, galaganda* and *kaphaja vyadhi.*

Special precautions: Reduce the dose in summer season.

Samirpannaga Rasa

Dose: ½–1 *ratti* (60–125 mg) bid with *madhu* or *ardraka svarasa.*

Indications: *Svasa, visuchika, adhyashana, pakshaghata, gradhrasi, katishula, ardhangavata, ekangavata* and *sarvangavata.*

Svarnavanga

Dose: 1–2 *ratti* (125–250 mg) bid with *madhu, makkhana* or *malai.*

Indications: *Svetapradara, shukrameha, sujaka, prameha, svapnadosha, viryadosha, shighrapatana* and *charma roga.*

Manikya Rasa

Dose: ½ *ratti* (60 mg) bid with *makkhana, mishri* or *madhu.*

Indications: *Rajayakshama* and *yakrita vikara.*

Svarnabhupati Rasa

Dose: ½–1 *ratti* (60–125 mg) bid with *madhu* or *ardraka svarasa.*

Indications: *Amavata, dhaturvata, shrinkhalavata, adhyavata, panguta, kaphavata, agnimandya, katishula, udavarta, grahni, ashmari, kustha, vidradhi* and *kshaya.*

Vyadhiharana Rasayana

Dose: ½–1 *ratti* (60–125 mg) bid with *madhu* or *ardraka svarasa.*

Indications: *Raktavikara, updansha, sandhivata, vatarakta, vrana, khalitya, nidranasha, netraroga, vrikkashotha, mushkavriddhi, shotha, shitapitta* and *nadivrana.*

Rasa-rasayana

Agastisutaraja Rasa

Dose: 1 tablet bid.

Indications: *Udarashula, kapha-vata vikara, shotha, shula, sangrahni, atisara, chhardi, sharkara, pittashmari* and *vedana.*

Agnitundi Rasa

Dose: 1–2 tablets bid.

Indications: *Dipana, pachana, vatanashaka, rasajirna, mandagni, yakrit-vriddhi, urdhvavata* and *kaphaja udararoga.*

Special precautions and contraIndications: *Uccharaktadaba,* children and *nutana vata vikara.*

It should not be used for long periods.

Ardhangavatari Rasa

Dose: 1–2 *ratti* (125–250 mg) bid with *madhu* and 500 mg of *trikatu churna.*

Indications: *Ardhangavata.*

Amira Rasa

Dose: 1–2 *ratti* (125–250 mg) keep in a capsule and then should be taken.

Indications: *Atashaka* and its *upadrava.*

Ashvakanchuki Rasa

Dose: 1–2 tablets bid

Indications: *Vatashula, kshaya, kasa, svasa, vali, palita, bandhyatva, katishula, sutika roga, dhanurvata, udara roga, yakrita-pliha vriddhi* and *kosthashula.*

Arshakuthar Rasa

Dose: 1–2 tablets bid.

Indications: *Arsha.*

Amavatari Rasa

Dose: 1 tablet bid with *madhu* or *ardraka svarasa.*

Indications: *Amavata.*

Arogyavardhini Rasa (Vati)

Dose: 2–4 tablets bid with *dugdha, punarnava* or *dashmula kvatha.*

Indications: *Shotha, vrikka vikara, antahsravi granthi vikara, prameha, kustha, rakta* and *mansa vikriti, mala sanchaya, vata-kaphaj roga, malavarodha* and *hridaya daurbalya.*

Note: It should not be used during pregnancy, *daha, moha, trishna, bhrama* and *pittadhikya.*

Icchhabhedi Rasa

Dose: 1–2 *ratti* (125–250 mg) at morning with cold water.

Indications: *Raktadosha, updansha, kustha, krimi, kaphaja jalodara, malavarodha* and *pakvashayagata mala sanchaya.*

Note: It is contraindicated in delicate person, children and pregnancy.

Updanshakuthara Rasa

Dose: 1 *ratti* (125 mg) bid.

Indications: *Updansha.*

Note: Sweet and sour food items, meat, milk and *kusmanda* should not be used while taking this medicine.

Unmadagajankush Rasa

Dose: 1 tablet bid with *brahmi ghrita.*

Indications: *Unmada, apasmara, mastiska daurbalya, murchha, yoshapasmara* and *anidra.*

Unmadagajakeshari Rasa

Dose: 2–4 *ratti* (250–500 mg) bid with *madhu* or *tambulapatra svarasa.*

Indications: As for *unmadagajankusha rasa.*

Ekangavira Rasa

Dose: 1–2 *ratti* (125–250 mg) bid with *madhu* or *vatanashaka kvatha.*

Indications: *Ekangavata, pakshaghata, ardita, gradhrasi, ardhangavata* and *dhanurvata.*

Karpura Rasa

Dose: 1–2 *ratti* (125–250 mg) with *madhu* or water.

Indications: *Atisara, pravahika* and *sangrahni.*

Kaphaketu Rasa

Dose: 1–2 *ratti* (125–250 mg) 4 hourly with *ardraka svarasa* and *madhu.*

Indications: *Kaphaja jvara, kasa, svasa* and *pratishyaya.*

Vrihat Kasturibhairava Rasa

Dose: 1 *ratti* (125 mg) bid with *ardraka* or *tambulapatra svarasa* and *madhu.*

Indications: *Sannipata jvara, shitanga, pralapa, tandra, nadi kshinata, sutika jvara, vishama jvara* and *visuchika.*

Krimikuthara Rasa

Dose: 2–4 tablets bid with *nagarmotha kvatha.*

Indications: *Krimi roga.*

Kamdudha Rasa

Dose: 2 *ratti* (250 mg) bid.

Indications: *Paittika vikara, raktapitta, amlapitta, atisara, shirah shula, chakkara, mastiska daurbalya, chittodvega, daha, murchha, bhrama, kshaya, urahkshata* and *mutrakricchha.*

Kamalahara Rasa

Dose: 1 *masha* tds with *takra.*

Indications: *Kamala, kumbhakamala, pandu, halimaka, shotha, mutrakricchha* and *raktavikara.*

Kaminividravana Rasa

Dose: 2 *ratti* (250 mg) at bedtime with *dugdha.*

Indications: *Shighrapatana.*

Kumarkalyan Rasa

Dose: ¼–½ *ratti* (30–60 mg) bid with mother's milk, *mishri* or *vacha* and *madhu.*

Indications: *Balashosha, balapakshaghata, hridaya-phupha-phusa-mastiska-gyanendriya-udara* and *vrikka vikara, akshepaka, kasa, svasa, kshaya, sangrahni, chechaka* and *motijharra.*

Kusthakuthara Rasa

Dose: 1–2 tablets bid with water.

Indications: *Kustha.*

Note: In case of burning sensation due to the medicine, *nagbala mula churna* with *madhu* should be given to the patient.

Gandamalakandana Rasa

Dose: 1 tablet bid with *kanchnara tvaka kvatha.*

Indications: *Gandamala, galaganda, apachi* and *granthi roga.*

Gandhaka Rasayana

Dose: 4–8 *ratti* (500–1000 mg) bid with *dugdha, mahamanjisthadi kvatha* or *khadirarista.*

Indications: *Kustha, raktaja vikara, shitapitta, dhatukshaya, prameha, mandagni* and *udarashula.*

Garbhapala Rasa

Dose: 1–2 *ratti* (125–250 mg) bid with *guduchi satva* and *madhu.*

Indications: *Garbhini vikara, garbhashaya daurbalya, garbhasrava* and *garbhapata.*

Grahnikapata Rasa

Dose: 1–2 *ratti* (125–250 mg) bid with *sveta jiraka churna* (1 *masha*) and *madhu.*

Indications: *Sangrahni, atisara* and *pravahika.*

Gulmakalanal Rasa

Dose: 1–2 tablets bid with *haritaki kvatha.*

Indications: *Gulma.*

Chaturbhuja Rasa

Dose: 1 *ratti* (125 mg) bid with *madhu.*

Indications: *Vata vikara, vali palita, jvara, apasmara, hastakampa, shirahkampa, sarvangakampa, kasa, shosha, mandagni, kshaya, yoshapasmara, jirnapakshaghata* and smooth muscles spasm.

Chaturmukha Rasa

Dose: 1–2 *ratti* (125–250 mg) bid with *triphala churna* and *madhu.*

Indications: *Kshaya roga.*

Chandrakala Rasa

Dose: 1–2 tablets bid with cold water, *dadimavaleha* or *ushirasava.*

Indications: *Paittika vikara, mutrakricchha, mutraghata, uccharaktadaba, raktapitta paittika prameha* and *raktapradara.*

Chandrakanta Rasa

Dose: 2–4 *ratti* (250–500 mg) bid with *madhu.*

Indications: *Shiroroga, ardhavabhedaka, suryavarta, jirna pratishyaya* and *anantavata.*

Chandramrita Rasa

Dose: 1 tablet bid with *madhu.*

Indications: *Paittika kasa.*

Chandranshu Rasa

Dose: 2 *ratti* (250) mg bid

Indications: *Garbhashaya dosha, yoni shula, yoni vedana, yoni daha, yoni bhransha, yoni kandu and yoshapasmara.*

Chintamani Chaturmukha Rasa

Dose: 1 *ratti* (125 mg) bid with *madhu* and *triphala churna.*

Indications: *Apasmara, unmada, pakshaghata, ardita, aptantraka, aptanaka, dandaptanaka, yoshapasmara, dhanurvata* and *akshepaka.*

Chintamani Rasa

Dose: 1 *ratti* (125 mg) bid with *madhu.*

Indications: *Hridaya roga, hridaya shula* and *hrid-drava.*

Jalodarari Rasa

Dose: 1 *ratti* (125 mg) bid with *ghritakumari svarasa, punarnava svarasa* or *dashmula kvatha.*

Indications: *Jalodara* and *shopha.*

Tribhuvankirti Rasa

Dose: 1 *ratti* with *madhu* and *ardraka* or *tulasipatra svarasa.*

Indications: *Navina* and *kapha pradhana jvara.*

Trivikrama Rasa

Dose: 1–2 *ratti* bid with *madhu.*

Indications: *Ashmari*

Trailokyachintamani Rasa

Dose: 1 *ratti* (125 mg) bid with *madhu.*

Indications: *Vata roga, snayu daurbalya, unmada, apasmara, aptantraka, visha, kshaya, kasa, svasa, sangrahni, prameha, jalodara, shula, shotha, hridya and rasayana.*

Nastapuspantaka Rasa

Dose: 2–4 *ratti* (250–500 mg) bid with *tila kvatha* and *gud.*

Indications: *Rajorodha.*

Nagarjunabhra Rasa

Dose: 1 *ratti* (125 mg) bid with *madhu.*

Indications: *Hridaya roga, arsha, hrillasa, chhardi, aruchi, agnimandya, shotha, amlapitta* and *raktapitta.*

Nityananda Rasa

Dose: 2–4 *ratti* (250–500 mg) bid with water or *gomutra.*

Indications: *Shlipada, kaphaja* and *vataja arbuda, apachi, gandamala, vatarakta* and *antravriddhi.*

Nidrodaya Rasa

Dose: 2 tablets at bedtime with water or milk.

Indications: *Anidra* and *vedana.*

Pratapalankeshvara Rasa

Dose: 2–4 *ratti* (250–500 mg) bid with *ardraka svarasa.*

Indications: *Prasutika jvara* and *sannipata.*

Pradarantaka Rasa

Dose: 1–2 *ratti* (125–250 mg) bid with *dugdha* or *amalki svarasa* and *madhu.*

Indications: *Pradara roga.*

Pramehagajakeshari Rasa

Dose: 1–2 *ratti* (125–250 mg) bid with *meshasringi kvatha* or water.

Indications: *Prameha, madhumeha, mutrakricchha, ashmari* and *daha.*

Pravalapanchamrita Rasa

Dose: 1–2 *ratti* (125–250 mg) bid with *anupana* as per *roga.*

Indications: *Gulma, pliha, anaha, udararoga, agnimandya, ajirna, udavarta, grahniroga, atisara, kasa, mutradosha* and *paittika vikara.*

Pandupanchanana Rasa

Dose: 3 *ratti* (375 mg) bid with lukewarm water or *gomutra.*

Indications: *Pandu, kamala, halimaka, yakrita vikara, pliha roga* and *kosthabaddhata.*

Piyushavalli Rasa

Dose: 1–2 tablets bid.

Indications: *Grahni roga.*

Puspadhanva Rasa

Dose: 1 *ratti* (125 mg) bid with *madhu.*

Indications: *Viryavikara, dhvajabhanga, shukrasrava, garbhashaya dosha* and *bandhyatva* of male and female.

Basantkusumakara Rasa

Dose: 1 tablet bid with *anupana* as per *roga.*

Indications: *Madhumeha, bahumutrata, prameha, napunshakta, somaroga, pradara* and *viryavikara.*

Bahumutrantaka Rasa

Dose: 2 *ratti* (250 mg) bid with *madhu.*

Indications: *Bahumutrata.*

Vrihat vatachintamani Rasa

Dose: 1 *ratti* (125 mg) tds–qid with *madhu.*

Indications: *Vata roga, anidra, yoshapasmara, hridaya roga, pakshaghata, ardita, dhanurvata, aptanaka* and *dandaptanaka.*

Vatakulantaka Rasa

Dose: 1 *ratti* (125 mg) tds-qid with *brahmi, shankhapuspi* or *jatamansi kvatha.*

Indications: *Apasmara, yoshapasmara, balapasmara, murchha, akshepaka, aptanaka, dandaptanaka, dhanurvata, pakshaghata, pralapa* and *chittavibhrama.*

Vatagajankusha Rasa

Dose: 1 *ratti* (125 mg) bid with *rasnadi* or *dashmula kvatha.*

Indications: *Vata roga, gradhrasi, krostukashirsha, avabahuka, manyastambha, urustambha, hanustambha* and *pakshaghata.*

Vataraktantaka Rasa

Dose: 2 *ratti* (250 mg) bid with 4 *masha sambhaga churna* of *neem patra, puspa* and *tvaka.*

Indications: *Vatarakta.*

Vantihrida Rasa

Dose: 1-2 *ratti* (125-250 mg) tds with *madhu.*

Indications: *Vamana* or *chhardi.*

Mahavatavidhvansana Rasa

Dose: 2 *ratti* (250 mg) bid with *madhu* and *mansyadi kvatha.*

Indications: *Vata roga, sandhivata* and *vatika shula.*

Vedanantaka Rasa

Dose: 1 tablet bid with lukewarm water or milk.

Indications: *Vedana* and *shula.*

Bolabaddha Rasa

Dose: 2–4 *ratti* (250–500 mg) bid with *mishri* or *madhu.*

Indications: *Raktapitta.*

Vrihat Vangeshvara Rasa

Dose: 1 *ratti* (125 mg) bid with *madhu.*

Indications: *Prameha, mutrameha, bahumutrata, shukrameha* and *viryadosha.*

Makardhvaja Rasayana

Dose: 2 *ratti* (250 mg) bid with *madhu* and *ardraka svarasa.*

Indications: *Shukra vikara* and *napunsakata.*

Manmatha Rasa

Dose: 2 *ratti* (250 mg) bid with *godugdha.*

Indications: *Napunsakata, shighrapatana* and *kamashaktihrasa.*

Mahalaxmivilasa Rasa

Dose: 1 *ratti* (125 mg) bid with *roganusara anupana.*

Indications: *Jvara, kustha, prameha, nadivrana, vrana, bhagandara, slipada, galashotha, antravriddhi, kasa, pinasa, pratishyaya, rajayakshama, sthaulya, daurgandhya, amavata, jihvastambha, galagraha, ardita, galaganda* and *shirahshula.*

Mutrakricchhantaka Rasa

Dose: 2–4 *ratti* (250–500 mg) bid with *mishri.*

Indications: *Mutrakricchha, mutravikara, mutraghata, ashmari, sharkara, vrikkashula, vastishula, tuni, pratituni* and *mutravrodha.*

Mriganka Rasa

Dose: 1–2 *ratti* bid with *madhu* and 10 *pippali* or *maricha churna.*

Indications: *Rajayakshama.*

Yogendra Rasa

Dose: 1 *ratti* (125 mg) bid with *madhu* and *ardraka svarasa.*

Indications: *Unmada, murchha, yoshapasmara, gradhrasi, pakshaghata, ardita, manyastambha, hanugraha* and *indriya daurbalya.*

Raktapittakulkandana Rasa

Dose: 1 *ratti* (125 mg) bid with *madhu* and *vasa* or *durva svarasa.*

Indications: *Raktapitta* and *paittika vikara.*

Rasaraja Rasa

Dose: 2 *ratti* (250 mg) bid with *madhu.*

Indications: *Pakshaghata, ardita, aptantraka, akshepaka, karnakshveda, antarayama, bahirayama, aptanaka, dantaptanaka, bhrama, chakkara, hanugraha, manyastambha, dhanurvata* and *raktachapa.*

Rasamanikya

Dose: ½–1 *ratti* (60–125 mg) bid with *madhu* or *makkhana* and *mishri.*

Indications: *Kustha roga, vatarakta, visarpa, vipadika, vicharchika, tvaka vikara, bhagandara, nadivrana, visphotaka* and *sveta kustha.*

Lavangabhraka Bhasma

Dose: 1–2 tablets tds–qid with water.

Indications: *Atisara, jirna grahni roga, pravahika* and *amlapitta.*

Lilavilasa Rasa

Dose: 2 *ratti* (250 mg) bid with *madhu.*

Indications: *Amlapitta* and *pitta vikara.*

Vrihat Loknath Rasa

Dose: 1–3 *ratti* (125–375 mg) bid with *madhu.*

Indications: *Yakrita* and *pliha dosha.*

Shashishekhara Rasa

Dose: 1 *ratti* (125 mg) bid with *erandamula kvatha* and *sunthi churna.*

Indications: *Andakosha* and *antra vriddhi.*

Svasakuthara Rasa

Dose: 1–2 *ratti* (125–250 mg) 4 hourly with *ardraka svarasa.*

Indications: *Svasa* and *kasa* (except *pittajasvasa* and *kasa*)

Note: It is also useful for insufflation in *shiroroga, murchha, yoshapasmara* and *ardhavabhedaka.*

Svasakasa chintamani Rasa

Dose: 2 *ratti* (250 mg) bid with *madhu.*

Indications: *Svasa* and *kasa.*

Shirahshuladivajra Rasa

Dose: 4 *ratti* (500 mg) bid with *godugdha* or water.

Indications: *Shirahshula, ardhavabhedaka* and *suryavarta.*

Shitapittabhanjana Rasa

Dose: 1–2 *ratti* (125–250 mg) bid with *madhu.*

Indications: *Shitapitta, udarda* and *kotha.*

Shothakalanala Rasa

Dose: 2–4 *ratti* (250–500 mg) bid with *talamakhana svarasa.*

Indications: *Shotha.*

Smritsagara Rasa

Dose: 1 *ratti* (125 mg) bid with *godugdha* and *brahmi ghrita.*

Indications: *Smritihrasa* and *smritidaurbalya.*

Sutshekhara Rasa

Dose: 1 tablet bid with *dadimavaleha* or *lajamanda.*

Indications: *Amlapitta, chhardi, gulma, mandagni, hikka* and *paittika vikara.*

Hinguleshvara Rasa

Dose: 1 *ratti* (125 mg) bid with *madhu.*

Indications: *Amavata.*

Hridayarnava Rasa

Dose: 1 tablet bid.

Indications: *Hridaya roga, hridaya daurbalya* and *hridaya shula.*

Vati-gutika

Chandraprabha Vati

Dose: 1–2 tablets bid–tds

Indications: *Prameha, mutrakricchha, ashmari, mutraghata, andavriddhi, pandu, kamala, halimaka, kustha, kasa, svasa, agnimandya, arochaka* and *rasayana.*

Dushivishahari Gutika

Dose: 1–2 tablets bid–tds

Indications: *Dushivisha, jangamavisha* and *sthavaravisha.*

Hinguvachadi Vati

Dose: 1–2 tablets bid–tds

Indications: *Hritaparshvashula, vastitrikayonipayu shula, gulma, vatavitmutrasanga, kantha bandha, hridgraha, pliha, arsha, hikka, adhmana* and *aruchi.*

Aptantrakari Vati

Dose: 2 tablets tds–qid with *maṇsyadi kvatha*

Indications: *Aptantraka* or *yoshapasmara.*

Arshoghni Vati

Dose: 2 *ratti* (250 mg) bid with *takra.*

Indications: *Arsha.*

Amavatari Vati

Dose: 3 *ratti* (375 mg) bid with *erandamula* or *rasnadi kvatha.*

Indications: *Arsha, gulma, shula, udararoga, yakrita-plihodara, pandu, kamala, aruchi, asthila, granthishula, gradhrasi, galaganda, gandamala* and *gudaroga.*

Eladi Vati

Dose: 1–4 tablets with milk.

Indications: *Kasa, raktapitta, chhardi, trishna, svarabheda* and *pittaja vikara.*

Karpuradi Vati

Dose: 1 tablet placed in the mouth and dissolve it five to six times a day.

Indications: *Mukhapaka, nukhadaurgandhya, dantavesta* and *jihvagata roga.*

Krimighatini Gutika

Dose: 2 *ratti* (250 mg) for adults and ¼–½ *ratti* (30–60 mg) for children with water or *madhu.*

Indications: *Krimi roga.*

Kankayana Gutika (Arsha)

Dose: 2–4 tablets bid with *takra.*

Indications: *Arsha.*

Kankayana Gutika (Gulma)

Dose: 2–3 tablets tds with lukewarm water.

Indications: *Gulma.*

Kutajaghana Vati

Dose: 2–4 tablets tds–qid with water.

Indications: *Atisara* and *sangrahani.*

Khadiradi Vati

Dose: 1 tablet 4–5 times a day.

Indications: *Mukhapaka, svarabhanga, danta roga, ostha roga, jihva roga* and *talugata roga.*

Guduchighana or Sanshamani Vati

Dose: 5–10 tablets 4–5 times a day with water.

Indications: *Jvara, daha, pittadhikya* and *trishnadhikya.*

Chandanadi Vati

Dose: 2–4 tablets tds–qid with water.

Indications: *Mutrakricchha* and *mutradaha.*

Chandraprabha Vati

Dose: 1–3 tablets bid with *godugdha, guduchi kvatha* or *gokshura kvatha.*

Indications: *Prameha, mutra vikara, viryadosha, andavriddhi, pandu, arsha, mtradaha* and *vrikka vikara.*

Chitrakadi Vati

Dose: 2–4 tablets bid with water.

Indications: *Aruchi, ajirna, udarashula* and *amatisara.*

Chhardiripu Vati

Dose: 2–4 *ratti* with *lajamanda* or *chandanadi arka.*

Indications: *Chhardi* and *utklesha.*

Takra Vati

Dose: 1 tablet bid with *takra.*

Indications: *Grahni roga* and *jirnatisara.*

Jatiphaladi Vati (sangrahani)

Dose: 1 tablet bid with *takra.*

Indications: *Sangrahani* and *atisara.*

Trailokya Vijaya Vati

Dose: 1 tablet bid with *madhu.*

Indications: *Pralapa, unmada, vrikkashula* and *kastartava shula.*

Dugdha Vati (Shotha)

Dose: 1 tablet bid with *godugdha.*

Indications: *Shotha.*

Panchatiktaghana Vati

Dose: 2–3 tablets tds–qid with lukewarm water.

Indications: *Vishama jvara.*

Pranada Gutika

Dose: 2–4 tablets bid with water.

Indications: *Arsha, pandu, krimi, udarashula, gulma, svasa, kasa, galagraha* and *hridaya roga.*

Plihari Vati

Dose: 1–4 tablets bid with lukewarm water.

Indications: *Plihavriddhi.*

Prabhakara Vati

Dose: 1 tablets bid with *madhu.*

Indications: *Hridaya roga* and its *upadrava.*

Vishamusti Vati

Dose: 1–2 tablets bid–tds with water or *tambulapatra svarasa.*

Indications: *Udara vata, udarashula, jirna vataroga, alarka visha* or *jalasantrasa, pakshaghata, ardita, kampavata, gradhradi* and *chestahrasa.*

Vyoshadi Vati

Dose: 1 tablet 5–8 times with lukewarm water.

Indications: *Pratishyaya* and *kasa.*

Vriddhibadhika Vati

Dose: 1 tablet bid with water or *haritaki kvatha.*

Indications: *Vriddhi roga.*

Brahmi Vati

Dose:1–2 tablet bid–tds with *makkhan, malai* or *dugdha.*

Indications: *Smritihrasa, anidra, murchha, yoshapasmara, unmada, pralapa, bhrama* and *hridaya daurbalya.*

Bhagottara Gutika

Dose: 1 tablet bid with *madhu* or *gojihvadi kvatha.*

Indications: *Svasa* and *kasa.*

Makardhvaja Vati

Dose: 1 tablet bid with *ardraka svarasa* and *madhu.*

Indications: *Dhvajabhanga* and *napunsakata.*

Madhumehanashini Gutika

Dose: 2–3 tablets tds–qid with *amalki* or *haridra svarasa.*

Indications: *Madhumeha* and *prameha.*

Rajahpravartini Vati

Dose: 1 tablet bid with lukewarm water or *ulatakambala kvatha* 7 days before the menstruation started.

Indications: *Rajorodha.*

Lashunadi Vati

Dose: 1–4 tablets bid with lukewarm water.

Indications: *Udara vayu, anaha, adhmana* and *mandagni.*

Sarpgandhaghana Vati

Dose: 1 tablet at bedtime with water or *godugdha.*

Indications: *Anidra, unmada* and *uccha raktachapa.*

Sabira Vati

Dose: 1–2 tablets bid with *godugdha* and *mishri.*

Indications: *Phiranga* and *upadansha* and their *upadrava.*

Note: Tablet should not be dissolved or chewed in the mouth.

Surana Vataka

Dose: 1–3 tablets bid with lukewarm water or milk.

Indications: *Arsha, vata-kaphaja grahani, kshaya, svasa, kasa, pliha, slipada, shotha, hikka* and *palitya.*

Sanjivani Vati

Dose: 1–2 tablets bid with *ardraka svarasa* or *madhu.*

Indications: *Jvara, sarpavisha, amadosha* and *mandagni.*

Sarivadi Vati

Dose: 1 tablet od at morning with *godugdha* or *raktachandana kvatha.*

Indications: *Karnasrava, karnanada* and *badhirya.*

Hingvadi Vati

Dose: 1–2 tablets bid–tds with *bhrista jiraka churna* and *takra.*

Indications: *Vatanulomaka, dipana, pachana* and *shulaghna.*

Parpati

Tamra Parpati

Dose: 1–3 *ratti* (125–375 mg) bid with *sukshma ela* and *bhrasta jiraka churna* .

Indications: *Yakrita vikara, pliha vriddhi, udara roga* and *sangrahani.*

Panchamrita Parpati

Dose: 1–3 *ratti* (125–375 mg) bid–tds with *bhrasta jiraka churna* and *madhu* and drink *dugdha* or *takra* thereafter.

Indications: *Sangrahani* and *jirna atisara.*

Sveta Parpati

Dose: 5–10 *ratti* (625–1250 mg) bid with cold water, coconut water or *takra.*

Indications: *Mutrakricchha, mutraghata* and *ashmari.*

Bola Parpati

Dose: 2–3 *ratti* (250–375 mg) bid with *madhu* and *mishri* or *durva svarasa.*

Indications: *Raktapitta.*

Lauha Mandura

Amlapittantaka Lauha

Dose: 1–2 tablets bid with *roganusara anupana.*

Indications: *Amlapitta, yakrita shula, trishna, mutradaha* and *pandu.*

Astadashanga Lauha

Dose: 1 tablet bid with *takra.*

Indications: *Kamala, halimaka* and *shotha.*

Guduchyadi Lauha

Dose: 2 *ratti* (250 mg) bid with *madhu* or *godugdha.*

Indications: *Vatarakta* and *raktavikara.*

Tapyadi Lauha

Dose: 3 *ratti* (375 mg) bid with *mulaka svarasa* or *gomutra.*

Indications: *Yakrita-pliha vikara, pandu, kamala* and *shotha.*

Tryushanadi Mandura

Dose: 1 tablet bid with *madhu* or *gomutra.*

Indications: *Pandu, shotha, udararoga, urustambha, kustha* and *pliha roga.*

Dhatri Lauha

Dose: 3–6 *ratti* (375–750 mg) bid with *madhu* before meal.

Indications: *Amlapitta, parinama shula, pakti shula* and *ajirna.*

Pradarantaka Lauha

Dose: 1 tablet bid with *mishri* or *madhu.*

Indications: *Pradara.*

Punarnavadi Mandura

Dose: 2–3 tablets bid with *punarnava svarasa* or *gomutra.*

Indications: *Shothayukta pandu.*

Balayakritari Lauha

Dose: 1 tablet bid with *madhu.*

Indications: *Yakrita* and *pliha vriddi, pandu* and *shotha* in the children.

Vishamajvarantaka Lauha

Dose: ½–1 *ratti* (60–125 mg) bid with *madhu.*

Indications: *Vishamajvara.*

Vidangadi Lauha

Dose: 4–6 *ratti* (500–750 mg) bid with lukewarm water.

Indications: *Krimi roga* and associated *pandu.*

Medohara Vidangadi Lauha

Dose: 1–2 tablets bid with *madhu* or lukewarm water.

Indications: *Medoroga, prameha* and *pandu.*

Saptamrita Lauha

Dose: 4–8 *ratti* (500–1000 mg) od–bid with *mahatriphala ghrita.*

Indications: *Netra roga* and *palitya.*

Avaleha Paka

Agastya Haritaki

Dose: 1 *harada* and *avaleha* bid with lukewarm water or milk.

Indications: *Kosthabaddhata, arsha, kasa, svasa* and *yakshama.*

Amritaprasha

Dose: 1 *tola* (10 g) bid with *godugdha* or *ajadugdha.*

Indications: *Rasayana, kasa, svasa, daha, trishna, raktapitta* and *shukrakshaya.*

Eranda paka

Dose: 1–2 *tola* (10–20 g) bid with lukewarm water or milk.

Indications: *Panguta, amavata, urustambha, shiragatavata, kativata, vastigata vata, kosthagata vata, vrishana vriddhi, shotha, udarashula, antrapucchha shotha* and *kosthabaddhata.*

Kantakaryavaleha

Dose: 1–2 *tola* (10–20 g) bid with lukewarm water.

Indications: *Svasa, kasa, hikka* and *kapha vriddhi.*

Kutajavaleha

Dose: 4–6 *masha* bid with *madhu.*

Indications: *Atisara, sangrahani* and *pravahika.*

Kusmanda Khanda

Dose: 1–2 *tola* (10–20 g) bid with *ajadugdha.*

Indications: *Raktapitta, kshaya, kasa, svasa, chhardi* and *trishna.*

Chitraka Haritaki

Dose: 6 *masha* bid with *godugdha.*

Indications: *Jirna pratishyaya, kasa, pinasa, krimi roga, gulma* and *udavarta.*

Chyavanaprasha

Dose: 1–2 *tola* (10–20 g) bid with *godugdha* or *ajadugdha.*

Indications: *Rasayana, kasa, svasa, trishadhikya, vatarakta* and *pittadhikya.*

Vasavaleha

Dose: 6 *masha*–1 *tola* bid with *madhu.*

Indications: *Raktapitta, kasa* and *svasa.*

Brahm Rasayana

Dose: 1½ *tola* (15 g) with *godugdha* or water.

Indications: *Mastiska daurbalya* and *smritihrasa.*

Haridrakhanda

Dose: 6 *masha*–1 *tola* (6–10 g) bid with water.

Indications: *Shitapitta, udarda, kotha, kandu, vicharchika* and *shotha.*

Guggulu

Amritadi Guggulu

Dose: 2–6 tablets bid with *guduchi kvatha* or lukewarm water.

Indications: *Vatarakta, kustha, arsha, mandagni, dustavrana, prameha, amavata, bhagandara, nadivrana* and *shotha.*

Abha Guggulu

Dose: 2–4 tablets bid–tds with lukewarm water or *godugdha.*

Indications: *Asthibhagna* and *asthishula.*

Kanchnara Guggulu

Dose: 2–4 tablets bid with *kanchnara tvaka* or *varuna kvatha.*

Indications: *Galaganda, gandamala, apachi, granthi* and *arbuda.*

Kaishore Guggulu

Dose: 2–4 tablets bid with *mahamanjisthadi kvatha.*

Indications: *Vatarakta, vrana, kustha, gulma, shotha, pidika* and *raktapitta.*

Gokshuradi Guggulu

Dose: 1 tablet bid with *gokshura kvatha.*

Indications: *Mutrakricchha, mutraghata, ashmari, shukradosha* and *mutradosha.*

Tryodashanga Guggulu

Dose: 2–4 tablets bid with lukewarm water or milk.

Indications: *Vata shula, sandhishula, pakshaghata, gradhrasi* and *vata vyadhi.*

Triphala Guggulu

Dose: 2–4 tablets bid with *triphala kvatha* or *gomutra.*

Indications: *Arsha* and *bhagandara.*

Panchatiktaghrita Guggulu

Dose: 6 *masha*–1 *tola* bid with milk.

Indications: *Kustha, nadivrana, arbuda, bhagandara, gandamala, gulma, arsha, hridaya roga, vidradhi, vatarakta* and *vataroga.*

Punarnavadi Guggulu

Dose: 2 tablets bid with *punarnavadi kvatha.*

Indications: *Shotha, jalodara, vriddhi roga* and *vatarakta.*

Panchamrita Lauha Guggulu

Dose: 1 tablet bid with milk or *erandamula kvatha.*

Indications: *Avabahuka* and *vata shula.*

Mahayograja Guggulu

Dose: 1 tablet bid with *roganusara anupana.*

Indications: *Vatavyadhi, amavata, sandhivata, ekangavata, sarvangavata, vatarakta, medovriddhi, nastartava, snayushula* and *udavarta.*

Lakshadi Guggulu

Dose: 2–4 tablets bid with *madhu.*

Indications: *Asthigata roga.*

Saptavinshati Guggulu

Dose: 2–4 tablets bid with *madhu* and *mahamanjisthadi kvatha.*

Indications: *Arsha, bhagandara, nadivrana, dustavrana, slipada* and *tvakavikara.*

Singhnada Guggulu

Dose: 1 tablet bid with lukewarm water and milk.

Indications: *Amavata, vatarakta, gulma* and *raktapitta.*

Churna

Astachurna

Dose: 2–5 g bid with lukewarm water.

Indications: *Mandagni* and *vataja gulma.*

Dadimadi Churna

Dose: 5–10 g bid with water.

Indications: *Vatakaphaja aptantraka.*

Dhatrinishadi Churna

Dose: 5–10 g bid with water.

Indications: *Prameha.*

Dviruttara Churna

Dose: 5–10 g bid with water.

Indications: *Shula, udara roga, anaha, visuchika, arsha, hridayaroga, gulma* and *urdhvavata.*

Guggulupanchapala Churna

Dose: 5–10 g bid with water.

Indications: *Kustha, bhagandara, gulma* and *nadivrana.*

Hinguvachadi Churna

Dose: 5–10 g bid with water.

Indications: *Hritaparshvashula, vastitrikayonipayu shula, gulma, vatavitamutrasanga, hridagraha, pandu, hikka, adhmana* and *arsha.*

Ajmodadi Churna

Dose: 3–6 masha (3–6 g) bid with *takra.*

Indications: *Amanubandhi vataroga,* i.e., *sandhishotha, amavata, gradhrasi, katishula, tuni-pratituni* and *visvachi.*

Avipattikara Churna

Dose: 3–6 g bid with cold water, milk or coconut water.

Indications: *Amlapitta* and *udarashula.*

Asvagandhadi Churna

Dose: 3–6 g bid with milk or water.

Indications: *Vata roga, mastiska* and *hridaya vikara, anidra, viryadosha* and *shukrakshaya.*

Karkatibija Churna

Dose: 3 g bid with lukewarm water.

Indications: *Mutrakricchha, mutradaha* and *paittika vikara.*

Kamadeva Churna

Dose: 3–6 g bid with *godugdha.*

Indications: *Vajikarana, kamecchhahrasa, shighrapatana* and *viryadosha.*

Vrihat Gangadhara Churna

Dose: 1–3 g bid with *madhu* followed by rice water.

Indications: *Atisara, pravahika* and *grahani.*

Chopchinyadi Churna

Dose: 3–6 g with lukewarm water or milk.

Indications: *Vrana, nadivrana, bhagandara, arbuda, vidradhi, upadansha, kustha, granthi, gandamala, galaganda* and *vatarakta* or *raktaja vikara.*

Jatiphaladi Churna

Dose: 1–2 g bid with water. Reduce the dose if mild sedation occurs.

Indications: *Grahani, atisara, pravahika, pinasa* and *pratishyaya.*

Talisadi Churna

Dose: 2–3 g bid with *madhu.*

Indications: *Shuska kasa* and *mandagni.*

Triphala Churna

Dose: 3–9 *masha* at bedtime with lukewarm water or milk.

Indications: *Kosthabaddhata, prameha, shotha, pandu, valipalita* and *netra vikara.*

Dadimastaka Churna

Dose: 3 g bid with *takra* or lukewarm water.

Indications: *Amatisara, agnimandya, aruchi, kasa, hritshula, parsvashula, grahani* and *gulma.*

Drakshadi Churna

Dose: 3–6 g bid with cold water.

Indications: *Amlapitta* and *chhardi.*

Dhatupaustika or Shatavaryadi Churna

Dose: 6–10 g bid with *godugdha.*

Indications: *Dhatukshaya* and *viryakshinata.*

Special precautions: It should not be given in case of *mandagni.*

Nagakesharadi Churna

Dose: 2–3 g bid with water.

Indications: *Raktatisara.*

Narayana Churna

Dose: 3–6 g bid with *takra.*

Indications: *Udara roga.*

Nimbadi Churna

Dose: 1–4 g bid with water or *giloya kvatha.*

Indications: *Vatarakta, kustha, tvaka* and *rakta vikara.*

Panchakola Churna

Dose: 1–3 g bid–tds with lukewarm water.

Indications: *Aruchi* and *agnimandya.*

Panchasakara Churna

Dose: 3–6 g at bedtime with lukewarm water or milk.

Indications: *Kosthabaddhata.*

Pusyanuga Churna

Dose: 2–3 g bid with rice water.

Indications: *Pradara roga.*

Balachaturbhadra Churna

Dose: 2–8 *ratti* (250–1000 mg) bid with *madhu.*

Indications: *Jvara, atisara, kasa* and *vamana* of the children.

Bilvadi Churna

Dose: 1–3 g bid–tds with water, *takra* or *dadima svarasa.*

Indications: *Atisara* and *pravahika.*

Mahasudarshana Churna

Dose: 3–6 g bid with lukewarm water.

Indications: *Jvara.*

Shivakshara Pachana Churna

Dose: 2–4 g bid with lukewarm water.

Indications: *Udara vayu, ajirna, kosthabaddhata, hikka, adhmana, anaha, aruchi* and *udarashula.*

Sarasvata Churna

Dose: 2–4 g bid with *goghrita.*

Indications: *Unmada, apasmara, mastiska daurbalya* and *smritihrasa.*

Sitopaladi Churna

Dose: 2 g bid with *madhu.*

Indications: *Svasa, kasa, kshaya, karapada daha, agnimandya, jihvastambha, parshvashula, aruchi, jvara* and *urdhvaraktapitta.*

Hingavastaka Churna

Dose: 3 g bid with lukewarm water.

Indications: *Ajirna, adhmana, agnimandya, udarashula* and *udara vayu.*

Hingvadi Churna

Dose: 2–4 g bid with lukewarm water or *takra.*

Indications: *Parsvashula, hridya shula, vasti shula, gulma, adhmana, anaha, grahni* and *svarabhanga.*

Hridya Churna

Dose: 1–2 *ratti* (125–250 mg) bid with *madhu.*

Indications: *Hridya vegadhikya* and *sarvanga shotha.*

Asava Arishta

Amalakasava

Dose: 15–30 mL bid with equal quantity of water.

Indications: *Prameha.*

Abhayarista

Dose: 15–30 mL bid with equal quantity of water.

Indications: *Agnimandya, arsha, grahani, pandu, kustha, udara roga, gulma, sopha, pliha, hridaya roga* and *chhardi.*

Amritarista

Dose: 15–30 mL bid with equal quantity of water.

Indications: *Jvara.*

Arjunarista

Dose: 15–30 mL bid with equal quantity of water.

Indications: *Hridaya roga.*

Ashokarista

Dose: 15–30 mL bid with equal quantity of water.

Indications: *Pradara, artavapida* or *kastartava, garbhashaya* and *yonibhransha, dimbakosha pradaha, yoshapasmara* and *bandhyatva.*

Ashvagandharista

Dose: 15–25 mL bid with equal quantity of water.

Indications: *Murchha, yoshapasmara, dhadkana, arati, chittavasthitata, chittabhrama, smritihrasa, shirahshula* and *manasika vikara.*

Ahiphenasava

Dose: 2–10 drops mix in water and drink.

Indications: *Atisara* and *visuchika.*

Ayaskriti

Dose: 15–30 mL bid

Indications: *Prameha, arsha, svitra, kustha, krimi, pandu* and *sthaulya.*

Ushirasava

Dose: 15–25 mL bid with equal quantity of water.

Indications: *Raktapitta, daha, mutrakricchha, usnavata* and *paittika vikara.*

Eladyarista

Dose: 15–25 mL bid with equal quantity of water.

Indications: *Visarpa, masurika, romantika, shitapitta, visphota, nadivrana* and *prameha pidika.*

Kanakasava

Dose: 15–25 mL bid with equal quantity of water.

Indications: *Svasa, kasa* and *urahkshata.*

Kalameghasava

Dose: 15–25 mL bid with equal quantity of water.

Indications: *Vishama jvara, yakrita* and *pliha vriddhi, pandu* and *kamala.*

Kutajarista

Dose: 15–25 mL bid with equal quantity of water.

Indications: *Atisara, sangrahani, raktapitta, aruchi* and *agnimandya.*

Kumaryasava

Dose: 15–25 mL bid with equal quantity of water.

Indications: *Yakrita-pliha roga, gulma, agnimandya, manda jvara, pandu udavarta, garbhashaya dosha* and *artava dusti.*

Khadirarista

Dose: 15–25 mL bid with equal quantity of water.

Indications: *Kustha,, kandu, dadru, raktavikara, granthi, vatarakta, visarpa, vrana, arbuda* and *gandamala.*

Chandanasava

Dose: 15–25 mL bid with equal quantity of water.

Indications: *Shukrameha, svapnadosha, mutradaha, prameha, pradara, upadansha* and *hridaya roga.*

Jambira Drava

Dose: 15–25 mL bid.

Indications: *Yakrita-pliha roga, gulma, asthila, arsha, udara-roga* and *medovriddhi.*

Takrarista

Dose: 15–25 mL bid with water.

Indications: *Arsha, grahni, jirnatisara, shotha* and *udara roga.*

Draksharista

Dose: 15–25 mL bid with equal quantity of water.

Indications: *Kasa, pratishyaya, kshaya, daurbalya, urahkshata, aruchi* and *agnimandya.*

Drakshasava

Dose: 20–40 mL bid with water.

Indications: *Grahani, arsha, pandu, kamala, daurbalya, kasa* and *raktaja vikara.*

Punarnavarista

Dose: 15–25 mL bid with equal quantity of water.

Indications: *Shotha, pandu, hridaya roga, udararoga, shakhagata vata, malabandha, hikka, kustha, kilasa, arsha* and *bhagandara.*

Balarista

Dose: 15–25 mL bid with equal quantity of water.

Indications: *Vatavyadhi.*

Vasarista

Dose: 15–25 mL bid with equal quantity of water.

Indications: *Kasa.*

Vidangasava

Dose: 15–25 mL bid with equal quantity of water.

Indications: *Udara krimi, vidradhi, urustambha, asthila, bhagandara, gandamala* and *hanustambha.*

Bhringarajasava

Dose: 15–25 mL bid with equal quantity of water.

Indications: *Dhatukshaya, rajayakshama* and *karshya.*

Mrigamadasava

Dose: 10–15 drops in 10 mL of water.

Note: In case of *shitanga sannipata,* 30 drops can be given by IV injection.

Indications: *Kaphaja sannipata, svasnishotha, hikka, vishuchika* and *shitanga.*

Mahamanjisthadyarista

Dose: 15–25 mL bid with equal quantity of water.

Indications: *Kustha, vatarakta, ardita, medovriddhi, slipada* and *raktaja vikara.*

Mustakarista

Dose: 15–25 mL bid with equal quantity of water.

Indications: *Atisara, sangrahni, ajirna, mandagni* and *udara roga.*

Rohitakarista

Dose: 15–25 mL bid with equal quantity of water.

Indications: *Pliha* and *yakrita vriddhi* and *shotha.*

Sarasvatarista

Dose: 10–20 mL bid with equal quantity of water.

Indications: *Manasika vikara.*

Sarivadyasava

Dose: 15–25 mL bid with equal quantity of water.

Indications: *Prameha pidika, upadansha, vatarakta, bhagandara, vrana, nadivrana* and *raktaja roga.*

Ghrita

Araghvadhamahatikta Ghrita

Dose: 10–20 g bid.

Indications: *Pittaja kustha, visarpa, daha, bhrama, gandamala, granthi, nadivrana, apachi, vidradhi, visphota* and *gulma.*

Brahmi Ghrita

Dose: 5–10 g bid.

Indications: *Vaka-svara-smriti-medha vikriti, unmada, apasmara* and *bandhyatva.*

Mahatriphaladi Ghrita

Dose: 6–10 g bid.

Indications: *Netra* and *drishti dosha.*

Durvadi Ghrita

Dose: 6–10 g bid

Indications: *Raktapitta.*

Panchagavya Ghrita

Dose: 5–10 g bid.

Indications: *Apasmara, kshaya, svasa, gulma, udara roga, vrishana shotha* and *panipada shotha.*

Panchatiktaand Mahatikta Ghrita

Dose: 3–6 g bid.

Indications: *Kustha, vrana* and *rakta vikara.*

Phala Ghrita

Dose: 6–10 g bid.

Indications: *Bandhyatva* and *napunsakta.*

Baladi Ghrita

Dose: 10 g bid.

Indications: *Hridaya roga.*

Mahachaitasa Ghrita

Dose: 3–6 g bid.

Indications: *Manasika* and *mastiska vikara.*

Taila

Amritadi Taila

Dose: External application

Indications: *Shiroroga, vatarakta* and *raktapitta.*

Anutaila

Dose: *Nasya.*

Indications: *Urdhvajatrugata roga.*

Irimedadi Taila

Dose: *Gandusha.*

Indications: *Mukharoga.*

Asaneladi Taila

Dose: External application.

Indications: *Netraroga, karnaroga* and *shiroroga.*

Astapatradi Taila

Dose: External application.

Indications: *Shiroroga, pinasa, kshavathu, karna* and *netraroga.*

Baladhatryadi Taila

Dose: External application.

Indications: *Raktamansabalakshaya, urdhvajatrugata roga, daha* and *shironetragata roga.*

Balaguduchyadi Taila

Dose: External application.

Indications: *Vatarakta.*

Bhringamalakadi Taila

Dose: External application.

Indications: *Andhya, badhirya, dantachala* and *svaravikriti.*

Chinchadi Taila

Dose: External application.

Indications: *Sarvangavata.*

Dhanvantara Taila

Dose: External application.

Indications: *Vata vikara, marmasthi roga, graha, antravriddhi* and *yoniroga.*

Dhurdhurapatradi Taila

Dose: External application.

Indications: *Khalitya* and *kandu.*

Erandashigruyadi Taila

Dose: External application.

Indications: *Karnanada, badhirya* and *karnashula.*

Karpasasthyadi Taila

Dose: External application.

Indications: *Vata vyadhi, avabahuka, pakshaghata* and *ardita.*

Ketakimuladi Taila

Dose: External application.

Indications: *Asthigata vata.*

Kottamchukaddi Taila

Dose: External application.

Indications: *Vata roga.*

Kshirbala Taila

Dose: Internal and external use.

Indications: *Asthigata* and *vataroga.*

Kumkumadi Taila

Dose: External application.

Indications: *Nilika, vyanga, vali, palita, tilakalaka, mukhadushika* and *varnya.*

Lakshadi Taila

Dose: External application.

Indications: *Balakshaya,unmaad, apasmara, papa, garbhini, yaksharaksha* and *bhutaghna.*

Malatyadi Taila

Dose: External application.

Indications: *Indralupta* and *arunshika.*

Madhuyastyadi Taila

Dose: External and internal application.

Indications: *Vatarakta, pittaja vikara, daha* and *ruja.*

Mahamasha Taila

Dose: Internal and external application.

Indications: *Pakshaghata, ardita, badhirya, hanugraha, karnanada, shirahshula, timira, kalayakhanja, pangu, gradhrasi* and *avabahuka.*

Mahanarayana Taila

Dose: External and internal application.

Indications: *Vataroga, ekangaroga, ardita, vepathu, pangu, badhirya, shukrakshaya, manyastambha, hanustambha, bandhyatva, kubjata, kshaya* and *jara roga.*

Nilibhrangyadi Taila

Dose: External application.

Indications: *Palitya, kampa, akshepaka, stambha, sosha, unmada* and *pinasa.*

Nimbamritadi Taila

Dose: External application.

Indications: *Sandhi-asthi-majjagata vataroga* and *kustha, nadivrana, arbuda, bhagandara, gandamala* and *arsha.*

Panchasneha

Dose: External application.

Indications: *Vatashula, stambha, bhagnashula, bahushosha* and *avabahuka.*

Pinda Taila

Dose: External application.

Indications: *Vatarakta.*

Prasarinyadi Taila

Dose: External application.

Indications: *Vataroga.*

Sahacharadi Taila

Dose: External application.

Indications: *Kampa, akshepaka, stambha, shosha* and *kativata.*

Unduru Taila

Dose: External and internal application.

Indications: *Gudabhransha.*

Kasisadi Taila

Dose: External application.

Indications: *Arsha.*

Kumbhi Taila

Dose: External application.

Indications: *Karnashula.*

Kustharakshasa Taila

Dose: External application.

Indications: *Sveta* and *audumbara kustha, vatarakta* and *kandu.*

Grahanimihira Taila

Dose: 3–6 mL orally with *ajadugdha* or *godugdha* and *abhyanga.*

Indications: *Sangrahani, udararoga, vali* and *palita.*

Chandanabalalakshadi Taila

Dose: External application.

Indications: *Daha.*

Panchaguna Taila

Dose: External application.

Indications: *Sandhivata.*

Bilva Taila

Dose: External application.

Indications: *Karnashula, karnanada* and *badhirya.*

Mahavishagarbha Taila

Dose: External application.

Indications: *Sandhishotha, gradhrasi* and *mansashosha.*

Vrihat Vishnu Taila

Dose: External application.

Indications: *Napunsakta* and *bandhyatva.*

Mahamarichyadi Taila

Dose: External application.

Indications: *Kustha, shotha, suptata, vrana, gandamala, granthi* and *udarda* or *kotha.*

Laxmivilasa Taila

Dose: External application.

Indications: *Mastiska roga*

Shothashardula Taila

Dose: External application.

Indications: *Shotha, slipada, vrana, nadivrana* and *dustavrana.*

Sadabindu Taila

Dose: External application(*nasya*).

Indications: *Shiroroga, shirahshula, suryavarta, khalitya, palitya, pinasa* and *pratishyaya.*

Vrihat Saindhavadi Taila

Dose: External application.

Indications: *Amavata, vata roga, andavriddhi, antravriddhi, sandhishula, ardita* and *ayama.*

Kshara Taila

Dose: External application.

Indications: *Karnashula, karnanada* and *badhirya.*

Kashaya

Aragvadhadi Kashaya

Dose: 15–20 mL mixed with 3 times water.

Indications: *Kustha, visha, jvara, chhardi, kandu, vrana* and *prameha.*

Araghvadhamritadi Kashaya

Dose: 15–20 mL mixed with 3 times water.

Indications: *Tvaka vikara.*

Ashtavarga Kashaya

Dose: 15–20 mL mixed with 3 times water.

Indications: *Vataroga.*

Balaguduchyadi Kashaya

Dose: 15–20 mL mixed with 3 times water.

Indications: *Vatarakta.*

Bharangyadi Kashaya

Dose: 15–20 mL mixed with 3 times water.

Indications: *Jvara, kasa, svasa, agnisada, hritparshvashula, shirograha* and *svayathu.*

Balashatavaryadi Kashaya

Dose: 15–20 mL mixed with 3 times water.

Indications: *Vata roga.*

Vrihatyadi Kashaya

Dose: 15–20 mL mixed with 3 times water.

Indications: *Mutra vikara.*

Chiruvilva Kashaya

Dose: 15–20 mL mixed with 3 times water.

Indications: *Arsha* and *bhagandara.*

Dashmulakatutraya Kashaya

Dose: 15–20 mL mixed with 3 times water.

Indications: *Vata roga, svasa, kasa, parshva-prastha—trika ruja, shirahshula* and *ansha ruja.*

Dashmula Kashaya

Dose: 15–20 mL mixed with 3 times water.

Indications: *Vata roga, kaphavata roga* and *sutika jvara.*

Dhanvantara Kashaya

Dose: 15–20 mL mixed with 3 times water.

Indications: *Vata vikara, sutika roga, kshina, marmasthi roga, antravriddhi* and *yoni roga.*

Dhanada Nayanadi Kashaya

Dose: 15–20 mL mixed with 3 times water.

Indications: *Ardita* and *akshepaka.*

Drakshadi Kashaya

Dose: 15–20 mL mixed with 3 times water.

Indications: *Vata-pitta vikara, madatya, chhardi, murchha, daha, srama, bhrama, urdhvaga raktapitta, pipasa* and *kamala.*

Elakanadi Kashaya

Dose: 15–20 mL mixed with 3 times water.

Indications: *Rajayakshama.*

Gandharvahastadi Kashaya

Dose: 15–20 mL mixed with 3 times water.

Indications: *Vata roga, kosthabaddhata, aruchi* and *managni.*

Guggulutiktaka Kashaya

Dose: 15–20 mL mixed with 3 times water.

Indications: *Sandhi-asthi-majjagata vata roga, nadivrana, arbuda, bhagandara, gandamala, pinasa, svasa, kasa, hridaya roga,mada, vidradhi* and *vatarakta.*

Kanashatavhyadi Kashaya

Dose: 15–20 mL mixed with 3 times water.

Indications: *Raktagulma.*

Mahamanjisthadi Kashaya

Dose: 15–20 mL mixed with 3 times water.

Indications: *Kustha, raktavikara, vatarakta, ardita, upadansha, slipada, supti, medodusti* and *netraroga.*

Maharasnadi Kashaya

Dose: 15–20 mL mixed with 3 times water.

Indications: *Vata roga, kampa, pakshaghata, avabahuka, gradhrasi, amavata, aptanaka* and *kubjatva.*

Nayopaya Kashaya

Dose: 15–20 mL mixed with 3 times water.

Indications: *Svasa* and *hikka.*

Panchkola Kashaya

Dose: 15–20 mL mixed with 3 times water.

Indications: *Gulma, pliha roga, udara roga, anaha, udarashula* and *mandagni.*

Pathyakashadhatryadi Kashaya

Dose: 15–20 mL mixed with 3 times water.

Indications: *Shirahshula, ardhavabhedaka, suryavarta, sankhaka* and *netra roga.*

Prasarinyadi Kashaya

Dose:15–20 mL mixed with 3 times water.

Indications: *Vataroga* and *avabahuka.*

Punarnavadi Kashaya

Dose: 15–20 mL mixed with 3 times water.

Indications: *Sarvanga shopha, uadara roga* and *pandu.*

Rasnasaptaka Kashaya

Dose: 15–20 mL mixed with 3 times water.

Indications: *Vataroga* and *jangha-uru-prastha-trika-prastha shula.*

Sahacharadi Kashaya

Dose: 15–20 mL mixed with 3 times water.

Indications: *Katigata vata roga.*

Trinapanchamula Kashaya

Dose: 15–20 mL mixed with 3 times water.

Indications: *Mutrakricchha.*

Vasaguduchyadi Kashaya

Dose: 15–20 mL mixed with 3 times water.

Indications: *Raktapitta.*

Varadi Kashayam

Dose: 15–20 mL mixed with 3 times water.

Indications: *Sthaulya.*

Adrikadi Kashaya

Dose: 15–20 mL mixed with 3 times water.

Indications: *Khanja* and *pangu.*

Balakulatthadi Kashaya

Dose: 15–20 mL mixed with 3 times water.

Indications: *Pakshaghata.*

Other Kalpa

Dashanasanskara Churna

Tooth powder

Indications: *Dantagata roga.*

Dashanga lepa

Lepa

Indications: *Visarpa, kustha, shotha* and *dustavrana.*

Pamari pralepa

Lepa

Indications: *Pama* and *kandu.*

Note: It should be started with minimal amount by mixing in *sarshapa taila.*

Use cautiously in delicate person.

Avalgujabijadi Churna

External application with *gomutra.*

Indications: *Svitra.*

Eladi Churna

External application.

Indications: *Visha, varna prasadana, kandu, pidika* and *kotha.*

Hribera kshara

External application.

Indications: *Svitra.*

Jadamayadi Churna

External application.

Indications: *Vatarakta.*

Kalaka Churna

External application as *kavala* and *gandusha.*

Indications: *Mukha, danta* and *gala roga.*

Kachuradi Churna

External application as *taladharana.*

Indications: *Shiroruja, buddhibhrama, hikka, netra roga* and *pinasa.*

Kolakulatthadi and Kottamchukaddi Churna

External application.

Indications: *Vata roga.*

Nagaradi Churna

External application.

Indications: *Shopha.*

Raktachandana Churna

External application.

Indications: *Vyanga.*

Upanaha Churna

External application.

Indications: *Vata roga.*

2 Therapeutic Index

Important

1. In this section, only names of the different medicinal preparations are given in accordance with the disease, so that there is a quick revision of different medicinal preparations available in the market for a particular disease.
2. Therefore, it is expected from the reader that they should observe first section of this book along with the relevant textbooks of the subject, so that the proper knowledge of the *matra* and *anupana* of the medicine can be obtained.
3. For composition of the medicine, it is necessary to observe the relevant textbooks of the subject as this book is merely a reference book only.

Sansthanagata

Pachana Sansthana

Medicines for *Amlapitta*

Kamdudha rasa, sutashekhara rasa, svarna sutashekhara rasa, madhuyasthi churna, amalaki churna, drakshadi gutika, amlapittantaka lauha, avipattikara churna, dhatri lauha, kapardika bhasma, pravala bhasma, muktashukti bhasma, shankha bhasma, chaunsathaprahari pippala, pravala panchamrita rasa, pittantaka rasa, piyushasindhu rasa, lilavilasa rasa, mahashankha vati, shambukadi vati, shankha vati, shulavajrini vati, kshudhavati gutika, lauha parpati and *triphaladi mandura.*

Medicines for *Atisara*

Agastisutaraja rasa, asvinikumara rasa, asvakanchuki rasa (jirna atisara), parpati kalpa (jirna atisara), anandabhairava rasa (jvaratisara), grahanikapata rasa, grahanigajakeshari rasa, pashupata rasa, vatebhakeshari rasa, bhuvanesvara rasa, lavangabhraka rasa, rambana rasa, kutajaghana vati, dadimapaka vati, dugdha vati (atisara), ahiphenasava, gangadhara churna, bilvadi churna, vyoshadi churna, lai churna, shatapuspadi churna, kutajarista, vatsakadi kvatha, takrarista, dhanyapanchakarista, mustakarista, dadimaputapaka and *dhanyapanchaka kashaya.*

Medicines for *Pravahika*

Dugdha vati (sangrahani), gangadhara churna, vrihat gangadhara churna, pravahikahara churna, dhanyapanchakarista, mahagandhaka rasa, lavangabhraka rasa, kutajaghana vati and *kutajarista.*

See *atisara* also.

Medicines for *Yakrita Vikara*

Tamra parpati, kalmegha navayasa, parpatadyarista, amavatari vati, balayakridari lauha, namakasulemani churna, arka lavana, kalmeghasava, tamra sindura, tamra bhasma, tamrachandrodaya, trivritta churna, kutaki churna, vrihat loknatha rasa, yakridari lauha, rohitaka lauha, rohitakarista, kumaryasava, plihari rasa, yakridaplihari lauha, agnitundi vati, asvakanchuki rasa, phalatrikadi kvatha, avipattikara churna, panchasuta rasa, chavyakarista, rasa sindura, svarnabhupati rasa, kamalahara rasa, trimurti rasa and *pandupanchanana rasa.*

Medicines for *Udarashula*

Shulaharana yoga, asvakanchuki rasa, anandabhairava rasa, aditya gutika, amavatari vati, shankha vati, mahashankha vati, shulavajrini vati, hingvadi vati, kshara vati, panchamrita parpati, avipattikara churna, hingavastaka churna, narayana churna, snuhi kshara, agnitundi vati, kravyada rasa, badvanala rasa, shulagajakeshari rasa, shulakuthara rasa, shulantaka rasa, shulanashana rasa, panchasama churna and *nidrodaya rasa.*

Medicines for *Antra vikara*

Lavangabhraka rasa, agnivardhaka vati, pippalyasava, aditya gutika, jirakadyarista, chaunsathaprahari pippala, dadimastaka churna, drakshadi gutika, drakshadi churna, panchakola churna, panchasuta rasa, tamra sindura, trivritta churna, amarasundari vati, mustakarista, dhatri lauha and *asvinikumara rasa.*

Medicines for *Kosthabaddhata*

Abhayarista, haritaki churna, sukhavirechaka churna, sakara churna, triphala churna, triphala guggulu, kutaki churna, haritakyadi guggulu, agnikumara rasa, ajirnakantaka rasa, naracha rasa, bhuvanesvara rasa, malashodhaka churna, avipattikara churna, saralavirechana churna and *trivritta avaleha.*

Kostha Shodhana

Icchhabhedi rasa, kampillaka churna, eranda taila, trivritta churna, panchasakara churna, trivritta avaleha and *aragvadhadi kashaya.*

Medicines for *Dipana* and *Pachana*

Agnikumara rasa, agnitundi vati, agnisandipana rasa, ajirnakantaka rasa, ajirnari rasa, badvanala rasa, gandhaka vati, chitrakadi vati, trikatu churna, shunthi churna, nagarmotha churna, ajmodadi churna, shatapuspadi churna, panchakola churna, kravyada rasa, dadimpaka vati, hingvadi vati, karpurasava, mustakarista, agnivardhaka vati, pippalyasava, aditya gutika, jirakadyarista, agnimukha lauha, agnimukha mandura, lavanabhaskara churna, hingavastaka churna, dadimastaka churna, kshudhavati gutika, panchamrita parpati and *dantyarista.*

Medicines for *Guda Roga*

Rasa sindura, vyadhiharana rasayana, agnisunu rasa, amritarnava rasa, arshkuthara rasa, arshoghni vati, kankayana vati (*arsha*), *pashupata rasa, piyushavalli rasa, piyushasindhu rasa, laghumalinibasanta rasa, pranada gutika, surana vataka, surana modaka, kshara vati, kasisadi taila, rasa parpati, shankara lauha, abhayarista, kutajarista, dantyarista, changeryadi gutika, changeryadi ghrita, pippalyasava, agastisutaraja rasa, triphala guggulu, panchasakara churna, avipattikara churna, jatyadi taila, vimala bhasma, gokshuradi churna* and *eladyarista.*

Hridaya evam Parisancharana Sansthana

Medicines for *Raktachapa Vriddhi*

Chintamani rasa, pravala chandraputi bhasma, mukta pishti, sarpagandha yoga, yogendra rasa, akika bhasma, akika pishti, mukta bhasma, javaharmohra, sangeyashaba bhasma, tagaradi kvatha, brahmi vati and *asvagandhadi churna.*

Medicines for *Hridayashula*

Nagarjunabhra rasa, hritachintamani rasa, prabhakara vati, sringa bhasma, gadamurari rasa, gulmakuthara rasa, chintamani rasa, vrihat purnachandra rasa, hingvadi churna, arjunarista, hingukarpuradi vati, mukta bhasma, pravala bhasma, javaharmohra and *sangeyashaba bhasma.*

Mutrala Aushadhi

Dugdha vati (*shotha*), *sveta parpati, punarnavadi churna, punarnavadi guggulu, parpatadyarista, punarnavarista, punarnavastaka kvatha, shothashardula taila, tala sindura, shothakalanala rasa, sudhanidhi rasa* (*shotha*), *kshara kalpa, trikantakadi kvatha, varunadi kashaya, varunashigru kashaya, durjalajeta rasa, asvinikumara rasa, panchatrinamula kvatha, mutrakricchhantaka rasa, ushirasava, svarnabhupati rasa, trivikrama rasa* and *mutrakricchhantaka rasa.*

Medicines for *Raktapitta*

Ushirasava, durvadi ghrita, vasa ghrita, kamdudha rasa, chandrakala rasa, chandrashekhara rasa, kaharvan vati, guduchyadi modaka, kravyada rasa, shankara lauha, madhukadya gutika, shilajatvadi lauha, sarivadi vati, bola parpati, raktapittantaka lauha, bolabaddha rasa, gokshuradi churna, kanakasava, muktapanchamrita rasa, raktapittakulakandana rasa, eladi vati, sutshekhara rasa and *svarnabasantamalti rasa.*

Medicines for Local Conditions

Abha guggulu, svarnabhupati rasa, lashunadi vati, trailokyachintamani rasa, navaratnakalpamrita rasa, sitopaladi churna, arvindasava, svarnabhupati rasa, dhatupaustika churna, bhringarajasava, mahayogaraja guggulu, saptavinshati guggulu, chopchinyadi churna, dashanga lepa, nirgundi taila, panchaguna taila, somraji taila, mahalakshmivilasa rasa, javaharmohra and *nagarjunabhra rasa.*

Medicines for *Hridadrava*

Nagarjunabhra rasa, javaharmohra, sringabhasma, pravala pishti, akika pishti, hridaya churna, arjunarista, hridachintamani rasa, mukta pishti, manikya bhasma, hritpatri churna and *sangeyashaba bhasma.*

Medicines for *Hridaya Vikara*

Arogyavardhini vati, kumudesvara rasa, chaturbhuja rasa, chintamanichaturmukha rasa, chaunsathaprahari pippala, javaharmohra, navaratnakalpamrita rasa, yakuti rasayana, arjunarista, hingvadi churna, pravalapanchamrita rasa, hridayarnava rasa, jambira drava, hritkapata rasa, prabhakara vati, mrityunjaya rasa, rasa manikya, chintamani rasa and *amritakalasha rasa.*

Svasana Sansthana

Medicines for *Kasa*

Panchasuta rasa, purnachandrodaya rasa, shilasindura, samirapannaga rasa, svarna bhasma, pravala bhasma, sitopaladi churna, abhraka bhasma, vasarista, amarasundari vati, kasakuthara rasa, kasakartari rasa, kasakeshari rasa, mahalakshmivilasa rasa, sringarabhra rasa, sringyadi churna, madhuyasti churna, sringa bhasma, talishadi churna, svasakasachintamani rasa, eladi vati, kanakasava, kasa vati, kasakartari gutika, lavangadi vati, agastyaharitaki, draksharista, vasachandanadya taila, bharangyadi kvatha, gojihvadi kvatha, bharangyadi avaleha, vasa avaleha, eladyarista and *khadiradi gutika.*

Medicines for *Svasa*

Somayoga, bhagottara gutika, panchamrita parpati, marichyadi churna, dhatura kshara, panchasuta rasa, kanakasava, somasava, rasa sindura, malla sindura, kaphakartari rasa, svasakuthara rasa, svasakasachintamani rasa and other medicines as indicated for *kasa.*

Other Medicines

Madhuyasthi churna, lavangabhraka rasa, guduchi satva, puskaramula churna, drakshadi gutika, haridra khanda and *shirishadi kvatha.*

Vatavaha Sansthana

Medicines for *Shula* and *Shotha*

Amavatari rasa, amavatari vati, hingulesvara rasa, svarnabhupati rasa, amritadi guggulu, tryodashanga guggulu, vatari guggulu, rasnadi guggulu, mahalakshmivilasa rasa, tribhuvanakirti rasa, vatavidhvansana rasa, mahavatavidhvansana rasa, trailokyachintamani rasa, vishamustyadi vati, saindhavadi taila, mahanarayana taila, vishagarbha taila, kshirbala taila, mahamasha taila, dhanvantara taila, prasarini taila, sahacharadi taila, karpasasthyadi taila, krishnachaturmukha rasa, vatagajankusha rasa, samiragajakeshari rasa, vatakulantaka rasa, rasnadi kvatha, maharasnadi kvatha, rasnasaptaka kvatha and *dashmula kvatha.*

Medicines for *Jvara*

Jvarankusha rasa, jvaramurari rasa, jvarari rasa, jvarashulahara rasa, jvarasanhara rasa, tripurbhairava rasa, tribhuvanakirti rasa, mahajvarankusha rasa, guduchighana vati, sanshamani vati, visvatapaharana rasa, mahajvarankusha rasa, mahanrityunjaya rasa, godanti bhasma, jayanti vati, jaya vati, sanjivani vati, sarvajvarahara lauha, mahasudarshana churna, mahasudarshanana ghana vati, amritarista, drakshasava, amritastaka kvatha, guduchyadi kvatha, patoladi kvatha and *panchabhadra kvatha.*

Medicines for *Avasada* and *Chinta*

Agastisutaraja rasa, unmadagajakeshari rasa, unmadagajankusha rasa, kumudesvara rasa, nidrodaya rasa, nidrodaya vati, sarpgandha ghana vati, asvagandharista, mansyadi kvatha, chintamanichaturmukha rasa, amarasundari vati, kamdudha rasa, chaturbhuja rasa, sarasvata churna, brahmi vati, sarsvatarista, samudradi vati, vatakulantaka rasa, akika pishti, akika bhasma, panchagavya ghrita, mahapanchagavya ghrita, kalyanaka ghrita and *mahakalyanaka ghrita.*

Medicines for *Chittodvega*

Brahmi vati, nidrodaya rasa, nidrodaya vati, vatakulantaka rasa, vrihat vatachintamani rasa, smritisagara rasa, chintamanichaturmukha rasa, amarasundari vati, sarpagandha yoga, rasa parpati, panchagavya ghrita, mahapanchagavya ghrita, mansyadi kvatha, kalyanaka ghrita, mahakalyanaka ghrita, sarasvata churna, sarasvatarista, asvagandhadi churna and *asvagandharista.*

Medicines for *Akshepaka*

Panchasuta rasa, tamra sindura, samirapannaga rasa, ekangvira rasa, suhaga, chaturbhuja rasa, vrihat vatachintamani rasa, vatakulantaka rasa, samiragajakeshari rasa and *amarasundari vati.*

Medicines for *Apasmara*

Rasa sindura (with *vacha churna* and *mansyadi kvatha*), *panchasuta rasa, tamrasindura* (with *mansyadi kvatha*), *amarasundari vati, kamdudha rasa, unmadagajakeshari rasa, unmadagajankusha rasa, chaturbhuja rasa, chintamanichaturmaukha rasa, trailokyachintamani rasa, vrihat vatachintamani rasa, samiragajakeshari rasa, panchagavya ghrita, mahapanchagavya ghrita, chaitanyodaya rasa, purana ghrita, sarasvat churna* and *sarasvatarista.*

Medicines for *Unmada*

Unmadagajakeshari rasa, unmadagajankusha rasa, akika pishti, akika bhasma, vatakulantaka rasa, vrihat vatachintamani rasa, samiragajakeshari rasa, ekangavira rasa, sarpagandha yoga, kalyanaka ghrita, mahakalyanaka ghrita, chintamani chaturmukha rasa, sarasvat churna, sarasvatarista, purana ghrita, tagaradi kvatha, mansyadi kvatha, trailokya vijaya vati, asvagandhadi churna, asvagandharista, brahmi ghrita, chaturbhuja rasa, dhatryadi ghrita, manasamitra vataka and *tungadrumadi taila.*

Medicines for *Ardhavabhedaka*

Chandramrita rasa, chandrakanta rasa, navajuvana rasa, shirahshuladivajra rasa, mahasugandhita taila, madhukadi hima, dashmularista, rasnadi guggulu, rasnadi kvatha, asvagandharista, nidrodaya vati and *pathyadi kvatha.*

Medicines for *Chakkara*

Svarnabhupati rasa, javaharmohra, kamdudha rasa, gadamurari rasa, mahamriganka rasa, laghvananda rasa, sutashekhara rasa, mansyadi kvatha, jatamansi churna, brahmi vati and *asvagandharista.*

Medicines for *Utklesha* and *Chhardi*

Agnikumara rasa, madhukadya gutika, eladi churna, eladi vati, rasa sindura, mayurapicchha bhasma or *mayurchandrika bhasma, pipalavriksha tvaka bhasma, agastisutaraja rasa, chhardiripu rasa, chhardiripu vati, nilakantha rasa, drakshadi kvatha, saptamrita lauha, sutashekhara rasa* and *panchamrita parpati.*

Medicines for *Kampavata* and *Gativibhrama*

Samiragajakeshari rasa, vatakulantaka rasa, vrihat vata-chintamani rasa, ekangavira rasa, kampavatari rasa, brahmi ghrita, kshirabala taila, mahanarayana taila, mahamasha taila, kaunchapaka, kaunchabija churna, vanari gutika, asvagandhadi churna, asvagandharista, chaturbhuja rasa, mansyadi kvatha, rasayana and *vajikarana yoga.*

Other Medicines

Ardhanarinatesvara rasa nasya, unmata rasa nasya, kamdudha rasa, gadamurari rasa, chaturbhuja rasa, vatakulantaka rasa, vatebhakeshari rasa, murchhantaka rasa nasya, kalakuta rasa nasya, sarvatobhadra rasa, malla sindura and *brahmi ghrita.*

Prajanana evam Mutravaha Sansthana

Medicines for *Mutradaha* and *Mutrakricchha*

Svarnabhupati rasa, chandrakanta rasa, chandraprabha vati, chandanasava, trivikrama rasa, mutrakricchhantaka rasa, gokshuradi churna, gokshuradi kvatha, sveta parpati, hajralyahuda bhasma, varunashigru kvatha, varunadi kashaya, kshara kalpa, parpatadyarista, sarivadyasava, gokshuradi guggulu, punarnavadi guggulu, basantakusumakara rasa, karkatibija churna, chandanadi vati, chandrakala rasa and *kamdudha rasa.*

Medicines for *Prameha*

Somesvara rasa, basantakusumakara rasa, pramehantaka rasa, abhraka bhasma, shilajatvadi vati, ayaskriti, vrihat vangesvara rasa, chandraprabha vati, madhukasava, dhanvantara ghrita, nishakatakadi kashaya, pramehagajakeshari rasa, vanga bhasma, svarna vanga, trivanga bhasma and *vastyamayantaka ghrita.*

Medicines for *Vrikkashula*

Varunashigru kashaya, varunadi kashaya, gokshuradi guggulu, hingvadi churna, kshara kalpa, mutrakricchhantaka rasa, kaharva vati, dashmularista, ushirasava, trikantakadi kvatha, asvinikumara rasa, nidrodaya rasa, nidrodaya vati, chandrakala rasa, pranada gutika, trailokyavijaya vati and *agastisutaraja rasa.*

Medicines for *Garbhashaya Dosha*

Svarnabhupati rasa, chandranshu rasa, navaratnakalpamrita rasa, ashokarista, lodhrasava, karpasarista, arvindasava, basantakusumakara rasa, manmatha rasa, puspadhanva rasa, phalaghrita, ushirasava and *shatpuspadi churna.*

Medicines for *Asthila*

Vrihat purnachandra rasa, parpatadyarista, varunadi kashaya, varunashigru kashaya, punarnavastaka kvatha, gokshuradi guggulu, kanchanara guggulu, chavyakarista, jambira drava and *vidangasava.*

Medicines for *Shopha*

Punarnavastaka kvatha, varunadi kashaya, punarnavadi guggulu, trikantakadi kvatha, trinapanchamula kvatha, shothakalanala rasa, punarnava churna, punarnavadyarista, dugdha vati (*shotha*), *punarnavadi lauha, punarnavadi mandura, shothari mandura, shothashrdula taila* and *sudhanidhi rasa* (*shotha*).

Medicines for *Ashmari* and *Sharkara*

Svarnabhupati rasa, chandrakanta rasa, trivikrama rasa, mutrakricchhantaka rasa, ratnagarbhapottali rasa, sveta parpati, hajralyahuda bhasma, varunadi lauha, varunadi kashaya, kshara kalpa, asmarihara kashaya, pashanabhedadi churna and *chandraprabha vati.*

Mansa, Asthi evam Sandhi Roga

Medicines for *Shula* and *Shotha*

Nidridaya rasa, nidrodaya vati, amavatari rasa, hingulesvara rasa, amritamanjari vati, mahayogaraja guggulu, singhanada guggulu, yogaraja guggulu, vatavidhvansana rasa, mahavatavidhvansana rasa, samirapannaga rasa, rasnadi kvatha, maharasnadi kvatha, dashmula kvatha, ajmodadi churna and *vrihat vaisvanara churna.*

Medicines for *Tantrika Vikriti*

Tryodashanga guggulu, amritabhallataka, ardhangavatari rasa, samirapannaga rasa, svarnasamirapannaga rasa, ekangavira rasa, chintamanichaturmukha rasa, vrihat vatachintamani rasa, rasaraja rasa, mahamanjisthadyarista, dashmula kvatha, dashmularista, maharasnadi kvatha and *vatagajankusha rasa.*

Medicines for *Shotha*

Agastisutaraja rasa, dashmularista, dashmula kvatha, shothakalanala rasa, shothashardula taila, mahavishagarbha taila, saindhavadi taila, kottamchukaddi taila, karpuradi taila and *guggulu kalpa.*

Antahsravi, Upachaya and Poshana Vikara

Medicines for *Upachaya*

Hemabhraka sindura, dhatupaustika churna, sitopaladi churna, asvagandhadi churna, shatavaryadi churna, hemagarbhapottali rasa, kshayantaka rasa, dashmularista, rasayana kalpa, vaji-karana kalpa, drakshasava, madhukadya gutika, muktadi vati, muktapanchamrita rasa, chandramukha rasa, agnisunu rasa, panchamrita rasa, veshvara, kshirabala taila and *mahamasha taila.*

Medicines for *Galaganda*

Shila sindura, gandamalakandana rasa, mahalakshmivilasa rasa, nityananda rasa, amavatari vati, kanchanara guggulu, mahayogaraja guggulu and *nirgundi taila.*

Medicines for *Prajanana*

Malla sindura, asvinikumara rasa, madanamanjari vati, kamagnisandipana rasa, vrihat purnachandra rasa, bas-antakusumakara rasa, manmatha rasa, makardhvaja vati, makardhvaja rasayana, vrihat vishnu taila, siddhavaradamrita rasa, navaratnakalpamrita rasa, arvindasava and *puspad-hanva rasa.*

Medicines for *Madhumeha*

Chandrakanta rasa, pramehagajakeshari rasa, basantakusu-makara rasa, vangesvara rasa, madhumehanashini gutika, vanga bhasma, trivanga bhasma, phalatrikadi kvatha, somesvara rasa, mehamudgara rasa, tapyadi lauha, chandrakala vati, shilajatvadi vati, sarivadi vati, devadarvyadyarista, pramehamihira taila, pramehahara kvatha and *chandraprabha vati.*

Medicines for *Asthikshaya*

Madhumalunibasanta rasa, svarnasamirapanbaga rasa, lakshadi guggulu, navaratnakalpamrita rasa, pravala bhasma, godanti bhasma, kapardika bhasma, muktashukti bhasma, shankha bhasma, muktapanchamrita rasa, kukkutandatvaka bhasma, abha guggulu and *puspadhanva rasa.*

Medicines for *Medovriddhi*

Jambira drava, mahamanjisthadi kvatha, medohara guggulu, navaka guggulu, ardhangavatari rasa, trimurti rasa, vatagajankusha rasa, medohara vidangadi lauha and *tryushanadi lauha.*

Medicines for *Raktalpta*

Agnimukha lauha, tapyadi lauha, kshayantaka rasa, shilajutvadi vati, parpati kalpa, agnimukha mandura, triphaladi lauha, punarnava mandura, lohasava, pandupanchanana rasa, mandura vataka, saptamrita lauha, manduradyarista, panchamrita lauha, panchamrita mandura and *dhatri lauha.*

Tvaka Vikara

Medicines for *Kustha*

Tala sindura (with *bakuchi churna, gomutra* and *khadirarista*), *shila sindura, svarnabhupati rasa, vyadhiharana rasayana, arogyavardhini vati, kusthakuthara rasa, kusthakalanala rasa, gandhaka rasayana, talakesvara rasa, rasa manikya, panchatiktaghrita guggulu, rasa parpati, kustharakshasa taila, tuvaraka taila, rasa sindura* and *panchasuta rasa.*

Medicines for *Shitapitta* and *Anurjata*

Vyadhiharana rasayana, haridrakhanda, sitapittabhanji rasa, somesvara rasa, astadashanga lauha, tapyadi lauha, shirishadi kvatha and *bharangyadi avaleha.*

Medicines for *Pama* and Other *Kshudra Kustha*

Rasa manikya, nimbadi churna, panchanimbadi churna, kaishora guggulu, amritadi guggulu, panchatiktaghrita guggulu, manjisthadi kvatha, mahamanjisthadi kvatha, sarivadyasava, marichyadi taila, mahamarichyadi taila, pamari lepa, khadirarista, svarna gairika and *gandhaka rasayana.*

Medicines for *Yuvana Pidika*

Gandhaka rasayana, kaishora guggulu, suddha svarna gairika, rasa manikya, nimbadi churna, panchanimbadi churna, puspanjana, haridrakhanda, tankana bhasma, manjisthadi kvatha and *mahamanjisthadi kvatha.*

Medicines for *Svitra*

Svayambhuva guggulu, udayaditya rasa, avalgujadi lepa, svitrari lepa, mahayogaraja guggulu, bakuchi churna and *bakuchi taila.*

Medicines for *Vrana*

Sarjarasahara malhara, jatyadi taila, jatyadi ghrita, saptavinshati guggulu, kaishora guggulu, panchatiktaghrita guggulu, sarivadyasava, manjisthadi kvatha and *mahamanjisthadi kvatha.*

Medicines for *Dadru*

Dadrughni lepa, kaishora guggulu, panchatiktaghrita guggulu, manjisthadi kvatha, mahamanjisthadi kvatha, khadirarista and *chakramardabijachurna lepa.*

Shalakya Tantra

Netra Roga

Vyadhiharana rasayana, saptamrita lauha, triphala churna, triphaladi ghrita and *chandrodaya varti.*

Nasa Roga

Anu taila, nasarshohara taila, sadabindu taila, mahamanjisthadi kvatha, rasa manikya and *kaishora guggulu.*

Karna Roga

Panchasuta rasa, sarivadi vati, rasaraja rasa, tryodashanga guggulu, asvagandhadi churna, badhiryanashaka taila, asvagandharista, kumbhi taila, bilva taila and *kshara taila.*

Mukha Roga

Irimedadi taila, khadiradi vati, jatyadi kvatha, rasa manikya, karpuradi vati, eladi vati, vyoshadi vati, vyadhiharana rasayana, kamdudha rasa, asvinikumara rasa (*mukhadaurgandhya*), *mahalakshmivilasa rasa, pranada gutika, sutashekhara rasa, sitopaladi churna* and *marichyadi gutika.*

Stri, Prasuti evam Balaroga

Garbhavastha

Indushekhara rasa, vrihat garbhachintamani rasa, garbhapala rasa, garbhavinoda rasa, navaratnakalpamrita rasa, arvindasava, sitopaladi churna, garbhavilasa taila and *srigopala taila.*

Prasutika Roga

Maghabra vati, saubhagya vati, dashmularista, mritasanjivani sura, dashmula kvatha, chaturmukha rasa, pratapalankesvara rasa and *devdarvyadi kvatha.*

Bala Roga

Chandrashekhara rasa, balajvarankusha rasa, kumarakalyana rasa, balarogantaka rasa, balarka rasa, rasapipari, arvindasava, shankhapuspi taila, sarvangasundara rasa, balajivana gutika, bala vati, muktadi vati, balachaturbhadra churna and *balagangadhara rasa.*

Other

Jaravyadhi

Rasayana yoga, tryodashanga guggulu, yogaraja guggulu, vrihat vatachintamani rasa, yogendra rasa, mahanarayana taila, kshirabala taila, mahamasha taila, gokshuradi guggulu, shankha bhasma, asvagandhadi churna, asvagandharista, balarista, parthadyarista, devadarvyadyarista and *akika pishti.*

Lasikagranthi Shotha

Shila sindura, gandamalakandana rasa, amavatari vati, nityananda rasa, kanchanara guggulu, panchatiktaghrita guggulu, mahayogaraja guggulu, kanchanaratvaka kvatha, navaratnakalpamrita rasa and *dashmula kvatha.*

Vrishana Shotha

Svarnasamirapannaga rasa, dashmula kvatha and *chavya-karista.*

Asthimajja Shotha

Vyadhiharana rasayana, lakshadi guggulu, abha guggulu, kukkutandatvaka bhasma, kapardika bhasma and *dashmula kvatha.*

Sujaka

Tala sindura, chopachinyadi churna, mahamanjisthadyarista, malla sindura, sarivadyasava, svarna vanga, amira rasa and *khunjunikari rasa.*

Antrakshaya

Tamra sindura, svarnabasantamalati rasa and *dashmula kvatha.*

Antrika Jvara

Amarasundari vati, vrihat kasturibhairava rasa, kasturi-bhushana rasa, javaharmohra, mahalakshmivilasa rasa, sutashekhara rasa and *bhunimbadi kvatha.*

Pratishyaya

Rasa sindura, samirapannaga rasa, kasturibhushana rasa, tribhuvanakirti rasa, guduchi satva, godanti bhasma, sanjivani vati, sudarshanaghana vati, sudarshana churna, dashmula kvatha, trailokyachintamani rasa and *panchavaktra rasa.*

Upadansha

Upadanshakuthara rasa, rasakapura, rasa manikya, somesvara rasa and *sabira vati.*

Svasni Shotha

Shila sindura, panchasuta rasa, samirapannaga rasa, svarna vanga, lakshmivilasa rasa, sringarabhra rasa, svasakasachintamani rasa, eladi vati, soma yoga, vyoshadi vati, lavangadi vati, sitopaladi churna and *kanakasava.*

Karna Srava

Panchasuta rasa and *sarivadi vati.*

Kukkura Kasa

Panchasuta rasa, manikya bhasma, pravala bhasma, sringa bhasma, pravala chandraputi, lauha bhasma and *talisadi churna.*

Antra Shotha

Svarnabhupati rasa, agastisutaraja rasa, agnikumara rasa, agnisunu rasa, kravyada rasa, dantyarista, mrigankapottali rasa, kshara vati, takrarista, dashmula kvatha and *grahnimihira taila.*

Masurika

Tribhuvanakirti rasa, brahmi vati (chechaka), eladyarista, sarivadyarista and *panchasuta rasa.*

Dhanurvata and *Dandaptanaka*

Panchasuta rasa, svarnabhupati rasa, rasaraja rasa, visnukrantamula churna (with *asvinikumara rasa*), *kalakuta rasa nasya* before and after of *ekangavira rasa, pratapalankesvara rasa, vrihat vatachintamani rasa* and *vatakulantaka rasa.*

Phuphaphusa Shotha

Rasa sindura, samirapannaga rasa, panchavaktra rasa, kalyanasundara rasa, vatebhakeshari rasa, mrityunjaya rasa, sringarabhra rasa, sringyadi churna, sringa bhasma, asvakanchuki rasa and *guduchi satva.*

Granthika Jvara

Kalakuta rasa nasya, lokanatha rasa, lavangasava, guduchi satva and *mahamrityunjaya rasa.*

Phiranga

Rasa manikya, malla sindura and *shila sindura.*

Rajayakshama

Tala sindura, manikya rasa, kumudesvara rasa, gadamurari rasa, rasa sindura, svarnabhupati rasa, chaturbhuja rasa, chandrakanta rasa, vijaya parpati, shilajatvadi lauha, yakshmantaka lauha, yakshmari lauha, mahamriganka rasa, svarnabasantamalati rasa and *sarvangasundara rasa.*

Visuchika

Tamra sindura, amritakalanidhi rasa (with *palandu svarasa*), *mrigamadasava, vrihat kasturibhairava rasa, basantatilaka rasa, grahnigajakeshari rasa, visuchikavidhvansana rasa, samiragajakeshari rasa, sanjivani vati, ahiphenasava, karpurasava, sutashekhara rasa* and *shankha bhasma.*

Visarpa

Rasa manikya, kaishora guggulu, mahamanjisthadyarista, nimbadi churna and *dashanga lepa.*

Suryavarta

Chandrakanta rasa, trikatu churna, guduchi satva, dashmula kvatha and *gadanti bhasma.*

Slipada

Nityananda rasa, slipadagajakeshari rasa, kaishora guggulu, mahalakshmivilasa rasa and *mahamanjisthadi kvatha.*

Rogavastha

Arsha

Rasa sindura, vyadhiharana rasayana, agnisunu rasa, amritarnava rasa, arshakuthara rasa, kravyada rasa, chaunsathaprahari pippala, pashupata rasa, piyushavalli rasa, piyushasindhu rasa, avipattikara churna, panchasakara churna, triphala churna, changeryadi gutika, changeri ghrita, chirubilvadi kashaya, kalyanaka guda, manibhadra guda, ratnagarbhapottali rasa, laghumalinibasanta rasa, arshoghni vati, kankayana vati (*arsha*), *pranada gutika, surana vataka, kshara vati, abhayarista, pippalyasava, takrarista, ktajarista, dantyarista, kasisadi taila* and *shankara lauha.*

Apasmara

Rasa sindura (with *vacha churna* and *mansyadi kvatha*), *panchasuta rasa* (especially in children), *tamra sindura* (with *mansyadi kvatha*), *amarasundari vati, kamdudha rasa, unmadagajakeshari rasa, unmadagajankusha rasa, chaurbhuja rasa, chintamani chaturmukha rasa, trailokyachintamani rasa, asvagandharista, brahmi vati, smritisagara rasa, hartala bhasma, manasamitra vataka, vatakulantaka rasa, rajata bhasma, basantatilaka rasa, vrihat vatachintamani rasa, samiragajakeshari rasa, sarasvat churna, sarasvatarista, purana ghrita, panchagavya ghrita* and *mahapanchagavya ghrita.*

Ajirna

Agnikumara rasa, hingvadi vati, agnitundi vati, agnisandipana rasa, ajirnakantaka rasa, ajirnari rasa, badvanala rasa, gandhaka vati, chitrakadi vati, dadimapaka vati, karpurasava, mustakarista, kravyada rasa and *sanjivani vati.*

Apachi

Shila sindura, gandamalakandana rasa, nityananda rasa, kanchanara guggulu, panchatiktaghrita guggulu, mahayogaraja guggulu, dashmula kvatha and *kanchanaratvaka kvatha.*

Ardhangavata

Ardhangavatari rasa, samirapannaga rasa, amira rasa, ekangavira rasa, yogendra rasa, brahmi vati, rasnadi guggulu, tryodashanga guggulu, mahayogaraja guggulu, dashmula kvatha, asvagandhadi churna, asvagandharista and *maharasnadi kvatha.*

Ardita

Rasaraja rasa, vrihat vatachintamani rasa, vatagajankusha rasa, svarna samirapannaga rasa, ekangavira rasa, chintamani chaturmukha rasa, dhatura kshara, mahamanjisthadyarista, mahamasha taila, kshirabala taila, prasarini taila, asvagandharista, asvagandhadi churna and *maharasnadi kvatha.*

Asthishosha

Samirapannaga rasa, lakshadi guggulu, abha guggulu, pravala bhasma, svarnabasantamalti rasa, lakshadi taila, kukkutandatvaka bhasma, kapardika bhasma, muktashukti bhasma and *kshirabala taila.*

Andavriddhi

Svarna samirapannaga rasa, vyadhiharana rasayana, chavyakarista and *dashmula kvatha.*

Agnimandya

Badvanala rasa, lavangabhraka bhasma, agnivardhaka vati, pippalyasava, aditya gutika, agnitundi vati, avipattikara churna, lavanabhaskara churna, chirubilvadi kashaya, drakysharista, hingavastaka churna, abhayarista, jirakadyarista, agnimukha lauha and *agnimukha mandura.*

Asmari

Mulaka kshara, varunadi kvatha, vastyamyantaka ghrita, vidangarista, chandraprabha vati, svarnabhupati rasa, chandrakanta rasa, trivikrama rasa, mutrakricchhantaka rasa, ratnagarbhapottali rasa, gokshura kvatha, varunashigru kvatha, sveta parpati, hajralyahuda bhasma, varunadi lauha, kshara kalpa, asmarihara kashaya and *pramehagajakeshari rasa.*

Asthivriddhi

Vyadhiharana rasayan.

Atisara

Agastisutaraja rasa, amritarnava rasa, asvinikumara rasa, asvakanchuki rasa (jirnatisara), anandabhairava rasa (jvaratisara), kanakasundara rasa, kamdudha rasa, grahnikapata rasa, grahnigajakeshari rasa, nrapativallabha rasa, pashupata rasa, puyushavalli rasa, vatebhakeshari rasa, bhuvanesvara rasa, lavangabhraka rasa, rambana rasa, laghumalinibasanta rasa, lakshminarayana rasa, hirnayagarbhapottali rasa, kutajaghana vati, dadimapaka vati, dugdha vati (atisara), ahiphenasava, gangadhara churna, vrihat gangadhara churna, bilvadi churna, vyoshadi churna, lai churnu, shatapuspadi churna, kutajarista, kutajavaleha, takrarista, dhanyapanchakarista, mustakarista, dadimaputapaka, dhanyapanchaka kashaya and *vatsakadi kvatha.*

Anidra

Agastisutaraja rasa, unmadagajakeshari rasa, unmadagajankusha rasa, kumudesvara rasa, nidrodaya rasa, nidrodaya vati, sarpagandha ghana vati, tagaradi kvatha, mansyadi kvatha, chintamanichaturmukha rasa, asvagandhadi churna and *asvagandharista.*

Aruchi

Agnisunu rasa, dashmula haritaki, dashmula rasayana, patoladi kvatha, sitopaladi churna, chaunsatha prahari pippala, vrihat purnachandra rasa, laghvananda rasa, sarvatobhadra rasa, kshudhabodhaka rasa, kshudhasagara rasa, kshudhakari gutika, panchamrita parpati, dadimastaka churna, drakshadi churna, lavangadi churna, panchakola churna, namakasulemani churna, shantivardhaka churna, jirakadyarista and *dantyarista.*

Amlapitta

Kamdudha rasa, kamdhenu rasa, gulmakuthara rasa, agnisandipana rasa, chandrakanta rasa, dhatri lauha, sukumara ghrita, shulavajrini vati, chaunsatha prahari pippala, nagarjunabhra rasa, piyushasindhu rasa, vrihat purnachandra rasa, vidyarabhra rasa, lavangabhraka rasa, lilavilasa rasa, sarvatobhadra rasa, sutashekhara rasa, drakshadi gutika, kshudhavati gutika, kshudhakari vati, panchamrita parpati, amlapittantaka lauha, madhuyasthi churna, avipattikara churna, drakshadi churna, shankha bhasma, kapardika bhasma and *pravala bhasma.*

Angadaha

Gadamurari rasa, guduchi satva, ushirasava, chandanasava, madhuyasthi churna, muktashukti bhasma and *pravala bhasma.*

Aptantraka

Chaturbhuja rasa, chintamani chaturmukha rasa, trailokyachintamani rasa, vrihat vatachintamani rasa, vatakulantaka rasa, yogendra rasa, sarpagandha yoga, aptantrakari vati, panchagavya ghrita, asvagandhadi churna, asvagandharista, sarasvatarista and *kalyanaka ghrita.*

Ardhavabhedaka

Chandrakanta rasa, navajivana rasa, mahasugandhita taila, anu taila, shadabindu taila, madhukadi hima, trikatu churna, godanti bhasma, pathyadi kvatha and *dashmula kvatha.*

Anantavata

Chandrakanta rasa, vrihat vatachintamani rasa, trailokyachintamani rasa, tryodashanga guggulu, shirahshuladivajra rasa, dashmula kvatha and *asvagandharista.*

Arbuda

Navratnakalpamrita rasa, nityananda rasa, kanchanara guggulu, lavangasava, nimbamritadi kvatha, shila sindura, guduchi satva and *dashmula kvatha.*

Antravidradhi

Guduchi satva, nimbamritadi kashaya, kaishora guggulu, saptavinshati guggulu, vyadhiharana rasayana and *navratnakalpamrita rasa.*

Asthila

Vrihat purnachandra rasa, parpatadyarista, varunashigru kvatha, gokshuradi churna, saptasara kashaya, rohitakarista, gokshuradi guggulu, kanchanara guggulu and *chandraprabha vati.*

Aptanaka

Vrihat vatachintamani rasa, vatakulantaka rasa, samiragajakeshari rasa, akika pishti, dashmula kvatha and *asvagandharista.*

Antarayama

Rasaraja rasa, vrihat vatachintamani rasa, vatagajankusha rasa, dashmula kvatha, maharasnadi kvatha, asvagandharista.

Avabahuka

Vatagajankusha rasa, samiragajakeshari rasa, tryodashanga guggulu, asvagandhadi churna, asvagandharista and *maharasnadi kvatha.*

Angajadyata

Ajmodadi churna, nagaramotha churna, vaisvanara churna, singhnada guggulu and *amritamanjari vati.*

Asthivikara

Lakshadi guggulu, abha guggulu, dashmula kvatha, muktashukti bhasma, kapardika bhasma and *praval bhasma.*

Amavata

Amavatari rasa, amavatari vati, svarnabhupati rasa, hingulesvara rasa, amritamanjari vati, triphaladi lauha, amritadi guggulu, singhnada guggulu, vaisvanara churna, ajmodadi churna, madhuyasthi churna, giloya satva, yogaraja guggulu, trimurti rasa, vrihat purnachandra rasa, vatavidhvansana rasa, siddhavaradamrita rasa, rasnasaptaka kashaya and *agnitundi vati.*

Atashaka

Tala sindura, chopchini churna, chopchinyadi churna, mahamanjisthadi kvatha, malla sindura, sarivadyasava, amira rasa and *khanjanikari rasa.*

Amashula

Panchasuta rasa, hargauri rasa, agnitundi vati, singhanada guggulu, kravyada rasa, chitrakadi vati, ajmodadi churna, piyushavalli rasa, vrihat purnachandra rasa and *lakshminarayana rasa.*

Akshepaka

Panchasuta rasa (in children), *tamrasindura* (with *svarna bhasma* and *jatamansi churna*), *samirapannaga rasa, chaturbhuja rasa, chandrodaya rasa, chintamanichaturmukha rasa, vrihat vatachintamani rasa, vatakulantaka rasa, asvagandhadi churna* and *asvagandharista.*

Antrakshaya

Tamra sindura, svarnabasantamalti rasa, pippali churna, dashmula kvatha and *drakshasava.*

Antrashula

Tamra sindura and *navajivana rasa.*

Amashaya karkatasphota

Tamra sindura.

Adhyavata

Svarnabhupati rasa, amritadi guggulu, yogaraja guggulu and *dashmula kvatha.*

Adhmana

Agnitundi vati, amarasundari vati, aditya gutika, navajivana rasa, vatebhakeshari rasa, hingvadi churna, hinguvachadi churna, panchasama churna and *vaisvanara churna.*

Antrika Jvara

Amarasundari vati, vrihat kasturibhairava rasa, kasturibhushana rasa, giloya satva, javaharmohra, mahalakshmivilasa rasa, sutshekhara rasa and *dashmula kvatha.*

Amatisara

Amritkalanidhi rasa, shambukadi vati, dadimastaka churna, bhunimbadi churna, sarvatobhadra rasa, gangadhara rasa and *mustakarista.*

Antravriddhi

Chavyakarista, nidyananda rasa and *vatari rasa.*

Aghata

Javaharmohra

Alasya

Panchavaktra rasa, asvagandhadi churna, asvagandharista and *dhatupaustika churna.*

Anaha

Pravalapanchamrita rasa, asvakanchuki rasa, changeryadi gutika, changeri ghrita, lashunerandadi kashaya and *yavakshara.*

Asragdara

Ashokarista, pusyanuga churna, muktapanchamrita rasa, durva ghrita, shatavari guda and *dhatryadi ghrita.*

Indralupta

Dhatturadi taila, nilibhringyadi taila and *malatyadi keram.*

Indriyashaithilya

Makardhvaja rasayana, makardhvaja gutika, vanari gutika and *kaunchpaka.*

Unmada

Samirapannaga rasa, chintamanichaturmukha rasa, amara-sundari vati, asvagandharista, brahmi ghrita, chaturbhuja rasa, manasamitra vataka, amarasundari vati, kamdudha rasa, unmadagajakeshari rasa, unmadagajankusha rasa, basantatilaka rasa, sarpagandha yoga, kalyanaka ghrita, mahakalyanaka ghrita, samudradi churna, dhatura kshara and *sarasvata churna.*

Udarashula

Shulaharana yoga, shankha bhasma ajmodadi churna, shatapuspadi churna, agastsutaraja rasa, aditya gutika, shankha vati, shulavajrini vati, hingvadi vati, kshara vati, panchamrita parpati, shulagajakeshari rasa, shulakuthara rasa, shulantaka rasa, shulanashana rasa, panchasama churna, hingavastaka churna, hinguvachadi churna, agnisandipana rasa, amritakalanidhi rasa, vidyadharabhra rasa, agnitundi vati, chitrakadi vati and *bhuvanesvara rasa.*

Urastoya

Rasa sindura, tala sindura, khanjanikari rasa, svarnabasantamalti rasa, naracha rasa, sringa bhasma, puskaramula churna and *dashmula kvatha.*

Urahkshata

Kusmandavaleha, sringa bhasma, dhatupaustika churna, rasa sindura, sitopaladi churna, madhuyasthi churna, kamdudha rasa and *abhraka bhasma.*

Udavarta

Svarnabhupati rasa, bhuvanesvara rasa, hingvadi vati, hingavastaka churna and *hinguvachadi churna.*

Udara Roga

Svarnabhupati rasa, agnisunu rasa, agnitundi vati, kravyada rasa, vrihat lokanatha rasa, narayana churna, vajrakshara churna, lavanabhaskara churna, jatiphaladi churna, shatpuspadi churna, hingavastaka churna, avipattikara churna, dadimastaka churna, hingvadi churna, abhayarista, chavyakarista, chittachandirasava, jambira drava, triphalarista, draksharista, parpatadyarista, mastvasava, lavangasava, chitrakadi vati, arka lavana, bhallataka rasayana, dashmula haritaki avaleha, dashmulapanchakoladi kvatha, draksarista, manibhadra guda, naracha rasa, jalodarari rasa, icchhabhedi rasa rohitakarista, saptasara kashaya and *sukumara ghrita.*

Udarda

Vyadhiharana rasayana, shitapittabhanji rasa, shirishadi kvatha and *haridrakhanda.*

Ushnavata

Asvinikumara rasa, asvakanchuki rasa and *kavabachini churna.*

Updansha

Updanshakuthara rasa, rasa kapura, rasa manikya, somesvara rasa, kaishora guggulu, sabira vati and *mahamanjisthadi kvatha.*

Urustambha

Vatagajankusha rasa, siddhavaradamrita rasa and *vidangasava.*

Ekangavata

Samirapannaga rasa, samiragajakeshari rasa, ekangavira rasa, tryodashanga guggulu, mahayogaraja guggulu, asvagandhadi churna, asvagandharista and *maharasnadi kvatha.*

Kamala

Kamalahara rasa, svarnabhupati rasa, trimurti rasa, muktapanchamrita rasa, pandupanchanana rasa, vrihat purnachandra rasa, murchhantaka rasa, somesvara rasa, dhatri lauha, kalyanaka guda, mandura bhasma, navayasa lauha, patoladi kvatha, yakritaplihari lauha, phalatrikadi kvatha, astadashanga lauha, tapyadi lauha, bhunimbadi churna, parpatadyarista, manduradyarista, kamdeva ghrita and *bhumyamalki kvatha.*

Kustha

Bakuchi churna, khadirarista, svarnabhupati rasa, vyadhiharana rasayana, arogyavardhini vati, kusthakuthara rasa, kusthakalanala rasa, gandhaka rasayana, talakesvara rasa, rasa manikya, panchatikta ghrita, nimbadi churna, kustharakshasa taila, tuvaraka taila, panchatiktaghrita guggulu, sarivadyasava, mahamanjisthadi kvatha, kaishora guggulu, ayaskriti madhukasava, madhusnuhi rasayana and *manibhadra guda.*

Kapha Roga

Rasa sindura, tala sindura, hargauri rasa, anandabhairava rasa, kaphakuthara rasa, kaphakartari rasa, kaphaketu rasa, kaphachintamani rasa, kalpataru rasa, durjaljeta rasa, mahalakshmivilasa rasa, slesmakalanala rasa, samirapannaga rasa and *kaphaghni vati.*

Kasa

Panchasuta rasa, purnachandrodaya rasa, shilasindura, samirapannaga rasa, abhraka bhasma, sitopaladi churna, vasarista, amarasundari vati, kasakuthara rasa, kasakartari rasa, kasakeshari rasa, kumudesvara rasa, chandrashekhara rasa, chandramrita rasa, vrihat purnachandra rasa, lakshmivilasa rasa, sringarabhra rasa, svasakasachintamani rasa, eladi vati, kanakasava, kasa vati, kasakartari gutika, lavangadi vati, agastyaharitaki, talisadi churna, draksharista, vasachandanadi taila, bharangyadi kvatha, gojihvadi kvatha, shirishadi kvatha, balajirakadi kvatha, bharangyadi guda, chitraka haritaki, chyavanaprasha, kantakaryavaleha, khadiradi gutika and *sringa bhasma.*

Karnapaka

Panchasuta rasa and *sarivadi vati.*

Kukkura Kasa

Talisadi churna, abhraka bhasma, sringa bhasma, giloya satva, panchasuta rasa, manikya rasa and *pravala chandraputi.*

Kaphaja Granthi

Tamra sindura, kanchanara guggulu and *kanchanaratvaka kvatha.*

Kastarajah

Kumaryasava, rajahpravartini vati and *tamra sindura* (with *sambhala bija, sauntha, elva, dalachini* and *kumaryasava*).

Kanthamala

Shila sindura, kanchanaratvaka kvatha, kanchanara guggulu, navratnakalpamrita rasa and *gandamalakandana rasa.*

Katistambha

Samirapannaga rasa, rasnadi guggulu, saindhavadu taila, dhanvantara taila, panchaguna taila, dashmula kvatha and *maharasnadi kvatha.*

Katigraha

Vishagarbha taila, mahavishagarbha taila, tryodashanga guggulu, singhanada guggulu and *dashmula kvatha.*

Katishula

Svarnabhupati rasa, vatari guggulu, tryodashanga guggulu, mahavatavidhvansana rasa, vatagajankusha rasa, maharasnadi kvatha and *dashmula kvatha.*

Kotha

Svarnabhupati rasa.

Kapha Vata Vikara

Agastisutaraja rasa.

Kosthabaddhata

Agnikumara rasa, ajirnakantaka rasa, naracha rasa, bhuvanesvara rasa, malshodhaka churna, sarala virechana churna, sukhvirechana churna, abhayarista sakara churna, avipattikara churna and *triphala churna.*

Kosthashula

Asvakanchuki rasa, anandabhairava rasa, avipattikara churna, hingavastaka churna, hinguvachadi churna, shankha bhasma, muktashukti bhasma and *shulaharana yoga.*

Krimi Roga

Krimikuthara rasa, krimimudgara rasa, krimighatini gutika, krimighna churna, vidangadi lauha, vidangasava, manibhadra guda, rasa kapura and *vidangarista.*

Kumbhakamala

Kamalahara rasa, bhumyamalaki kvatha, phalatrikadi kvatha and *rohitakarista.*

Kampavata

Kalakuta rasa nasya, samiragajakeshari rasa, kampavatari rasa and *vatari gutika.*

Kamonmattata

Chandrodaya rasa.

Krostukashirsha

Vatagajankusha rasa and *dashmula kvatha.*

Kamjori

Makardhvaja rasayana, makardhvaja gutika, mushalipaka, balarista and *dhatupaustika churna.*

Karnanada

Rasaraja rasa, tryodashanga guggulu, dashmula kvatha, maharasnadi kvatha, asvagandhadi churna and *asvagandharista.*

Karnasrava

Sarivadi vati, dashmula kvatha and *kapardika bhasma.*

Karnaroga

Sarivadi vati, kumbhi taila, bilva taila, kshara taila, asanavilvadi taila and *vachalashunadi taila.*

Kaphatisara

Lokanatha rasa, trikatu churna, chitrakadi vati and *mustakarista.*

Kubjatva

Samiragajakeshari rasa, dashmula kvatha, balarista and *asvagandhadi churna.*

Kandu

Somesvara rasa, astangadashanga lauha, tapyadi lauha, chandanabalalakshadi taila, haridra khanda, gandhakapishti taila and *mahamarichyadi taila.*

Karshya

Karshyahara lauha, shatavari churna, sitopaladi churna, arvindasava, balarista, asvagandharista, kshirabala taila, mahamasha taila, drakshasava, vidaryadi ghrita and *dhatu-paustika churna.*

Kosthavikara

Abhaya lavana and *narikela lavana.*

Khalli

Tamra sindura, pratapalankesvara rasa, dashmula kvatha, maharasnadi kvatha, asvagandhadi churna and *mahayogaraja guggulu.*

Khalitya

Vyadhiharana rasayana, bhringaraja taila, mahabhringaraja taila, nilibhrangyadi taila, dhutturadi taila and *triphaladya taila.*

Keshapata

Nilibhrangyadi taila, bhrangamalakadi taila, dhutturadi taila and *shadabindu taila nasya.*

Khanjavata

Samiragajakeshari rasa, mahayograja guggulu, singhanada guggulu, tryodashanga guggulu, vrihat vatachintamani rasa and *maharasnadi kvatha.*

Khanja

Prasarinyadi taila, vatari guggulu, tryodashanga guggulu, vrihat vatachintamani rasa, asvagandharista, mahavatavidhvansana rasa and *maharasnadi kvatha.*

Kastartava

Kasisa bhasma and *rajahpravartini vati.*

See *kastarajaha* also.

Kilasa

Madhukasava, mahamanjisthadi kvatha, kaishora guggulu, patoladi kvatha, khadirarista and *madhusnuhi rasayana.*

Gudabhransha

Agastisutaraja rasa, changeryadi ghrita, pippalyadi ghrita and *mushakadi taila.*

Gulma

Hingvadi churna, svarnabhupati rasa, rasa sindura, tamra sindura, trimurti rasa, agnikumara rasa, kshara vati, agnisandipana rasa, kravyada rasa, kankayana vati (gulma), gulmakalanala rasa, gulmakuthara rasa, naracha rasa, pravalapanchamrita rasa, badvanala rasa, mahamriganka rasa, somesvara rasa, amavatari vati, ksharakalpa, chavyakarista, jambira drava, parpatadyarista and *vidangasava.*

Galaganda

Shila sindura, gandamalakandana rasa, mahalakshmivilasa rasa, nityananda rasa, nirgundi taila, amavatari vati, kanchanara guggulu, mahayogaraja guggulu and *kanchanaratvaka kvatha.*

Gradhrasi

Vatari guggulu, tryodashanga guggulu, rasnadi guggulu, vrihat vatachintamani rasa, mahavatavidhvansana rasa, samirapannaga rasa, mahavishagarbha taila, prasarinyadi taila, sahacharadi taila, ekangavira rasa, vatagajankusha rasa, samiragajakeshari rasa, asvagandhadi churna, asvagandharista and *maharasnadi kvatha.*

Grahani

Svarnabhupati rasa, agastisutaraja rasa, agnikumara rasa, agnisunu rasa, kravyada rasa, dantyarista, mrigankapottali rasa, lavanabhaskara churna, vrihat gangadhara rasa, changeryadi gutika, changeryadi ghrita, hingavastaka churna, grahnikapata rasa, jirakadyarista, mustakarista, shankha bhasma, kapardika bhasma, kukkutandatvaka bhasma, muktashukti bhasma, kutaja ghanavati, kutajarista, kutajavaleha, panchamrita parpati, piyushavalli rasa kshara vati, takrarista and *grahnimihira taila.*

Garbhashayadusti

Svarnabhupati rasa, chandransu rasa, navaratnakalpamrita rasa, ashokarista and *karpasarista.*

Gulma Vedana

Amritarnava rasa and *agastisutaraja rasa.*

Garbhini Roga

Indushekhara rasa, vrihat garbhachintamani rasa, garbhapala rasa and *garbhavinoda rasa.*

Granthika Sannipata

Kalakuta rasa, lokanatha rasa and *lavangasava.*

Gandamala

Gandamalakandana rasa, nityananda rasa, amavatari vati, svarnabasantamalti rasa, kanchanara guggulu, mahayogaraja guggulu, vidangasava and *nirgundi taila.*

Garbhashaya Shosha

Navaratnakalpamrita rasa, arvindasava and *sitopaladi churna.*

Garbhashaya Vikara

Basantakusumakara rasa and *manmatha rasa.*

Galagraha

Mahalakshmivilasa rasa, pranada gutika, talisadi churna and *dashmula kvatha.*

Granthi Roga

Lokanatha rasa, lavangasava, kanchanara guggulu, mahayogaraja guggulu, chopachinyadi churna and *nirgundi taila.*

Granthishula

Amavatari vati.

Garbhashula

Garbhavilasa taila.

See *garbhini roga* also.

Ghabrahata

Javaharmohra, arjunarista and *prabhakara vati.*

Charma Vikara

Shila sindura, nimbadi churna, panchanimbadi churna, kaishora guggulu, panchatiktaghrita guggulu, marichyadi taila, karanja taila, tuvaraka taila, sarshapadi taila, khadirarista, sarivadyasava, manjisthadi kvatha and *mahamanjisthadi kvatha.*

Chakkara

Svarnabhupati rasa, asvagandharista, asvagandhadi churna and *kamdudha rasa.*

Chechaka

Tribhuvanakirti rasa, brahmi vati (*chechaka*)and *eladyarista.*

Chittavibhrama

Vatakulantaka rasa, vrihat vatachintamani rasa, trailokya-chintamani rasa, asvagandhadi churna, asvagandharista, brahmi vati, brahmi ghrita, panchagavya ghrita and *mahapan-chagavya ghrita.*

Chhardi

Agnikumara rasa, madhukadya gutika, eladi churna, eladi vati, drakshadi kvatha, saptamrita lauha, mayurapicchha bhasma, vantihrada rasa and *sutashekhara rasa.*

Jirna Jvara

Patoladi kvatha, amritarista, sanshamani vati, giloya satva, asvinikumara rasa, kamdudha rasa, kamdhenu rasa kumudesvara rasa, gadamurari rasa, jayamangala rasa, jirnajvarankusha rasa, vidyadharabhra rasa, madhumalinibasanta rasa, muktapanchamrita rasa, mahamriganka rasa and *kshayantaka rasa.*

Jantughna

Tala sindura.

Jalodara

Durjalajeta rasa, vijaya parpati, tala sindura, tamra sindura, jalodarari rasa, navaratnakalpamrita rasa, punarnavadi guggulu, gokshuradi guggulu, punarnavastaka kvatha and *punarnavarista.*

Jvara

Amritarista, sudarshana churna, sudarshana ghanavati, sanshamani vati, giloya satva, patoladi kvatha, svarnabhupati rasa, svarnasindura, hargauri rasa, agnisunu rasa, ardhanarinatesvara rasa nasya, amritkalanidhi rasa, asvinikumara rasa, kasturibhairava rasa, gadamurari rasa (dhatugata jvara), jvarankusha rasa, jvaramurari rasa, jvarari rasa, jvarashulahara rasa, jvarasanhara rasa, jvarakeshari rasa, tripurabhairava rasa, tribhuvanakirti rasa, narayanajvarankusha rasa (sannipata jvara), visvatapaharana rasa, betala rasa, mahajvarankusha rasa, mahamrityunjaya rasa, mrityunjaya rasa, ratnagiri rasa, laghumalinibasanta rasa, svacchhandabhairava rasa, svarnabasantamalti rasa, hingulesvara rasa, guduchi ghana vati, jayanti vati, jaya vati, navajvarahara vati, sanjivani vati, hingukarpuradi vati, malla parpati, chandanadi lauha, sarvajvarahara lauha, mahasudarshana churna, drakshasava, kiratadi taila, mahalakshadi taila, chandanabalalakshadi taila, amritastaka kvatha, guduchyadi kvatha and *panchabhadra kvatha.*

Tandra

Malla sindura, panchavaktra rasa, ardhanarinatesvara rasa nasya and *kalakuta rasa nasya.*

Tamaka Svasa

Svarnasamirapannaga rasa, malla sindura, svasahara kashaya, balajirakadi kvatha and *svasakuthara rasa.*

See *svasa* also.

Trishna

Gadamurari rasa, lilavilasa rasa, eladi churna, kumkumadi churna and *shadangapaniya.*

Tvaka Vikara

Gandhaka rasayana, khadirarista, kasisadi ghrita and *viparitamall taila.*

See *charma vikara* also.

Tapa

Rasadi rasa, muktashukti bhasma, mukta bhasma and *mukta pishti.*

Dantodabheda

Panchasuta rasa, kanakasundara rasa and *dantodabhedagadantaka rasa.*

Daha

Agastisutaraja rasa, kamdudha rasa, guduchyadi modaka, chandrakala rasa, pramehagajakesari rasa, rasadi rasa, lilavilasa rasa, kaharvan vati, chandanadi lauha and *nagakesharadi churna.*

Dadru

Devdarvarista, haridra khanda, kasisadi ghrita and *dadrughni lepa.*

Dandaptanaka

Chintamanichaturmukha rasa, vrihat vatachintamani rasa and *vatakulantaka rasa.*

Daurbalya

Murchhantaka rasa, mrigankapottali rasa, kamalalakshadi churna, dhatupaustika churna, sitopaladi churna, draksharista, drakshasava, phalarista, mahachandanadi taila, svarnabasantamalti rasa and *shatavari churna.*

Dusta Vrana

Rasa kapura.

Danta Roga

Karpuradi vati, dashanasanskara churna, irimedadi taila and *khadiradi vati.*

Dhanurvata

Panchasuta rasa (especially in children)*, svarnabhupati rasa, rasaraja rasa, visnukrantamula churna* (with *asvakanchuki rasa*)*, kalakuta rasa nasya* before and after giving *ekangavira, chandrodaya rasa, chintamanichaturmukha rasa, pratapalankesvara rasa, vrihat vatachintamani rasa, vatakulantaka rasa, dashmula kvatha* and *maharasnadi kvatha.*

Dhanustankara

Khanjanikari rasa and *lakshminarayana rasa.*

Dhvajabhanga

Kamdhenu rasa, chandrakanta rasa, puspadhanva rasa, vanari gutika, kapikacchhubija churna, makardhvaja rasayana, makardhvaja gutika, asvagandhadi churna, kaunchapaka, manmatha rasa and *kamchudamani rasa.*

Dhadkana

Kumudesvara rasa, chintamani rasa, nagarjunabhra rasa, prabhakara vati and *javaharmohra.*

Dhatuvisha

Gandhaka rasayana and *amalki churna.*

Dhatukshaya

Dhatupaustika churna, shatavari churna, asvagandhadi churna, balarista, drakshasava, angurasava, asvagandharista, arvindasava and *bhringarajasava.*

Navajvara

Godantihartala bhasma, hingulesvara rasa, sanjivani vati, sudarshana churna, sudarshana ghanavati and *patoladi kvatha.*

See *jvara* also.

Niruddhaprakasha

Panchasuta rasa.

Napunsakta

Malla sindura, asvinikumara rasa, madanamanjari vati, kamagnisandipana rasa, vrihat purnachandra rasa, basantakusumakara rasa, manmatha rasa, makardhvaja vati, vrihat visnu taila and *kaunchapaka avaleha.*

Nasa Vrana

Vyadhiharana rasayana, saptavinshati guggulu, kaishora guggulu, mahamanjisthadi kvatha, manjisthadyarista, sarivadyasava and *nimbadi churna.*

Nadivrana

Vyadhiharana rasayana, rasa kapura, hartala bhasma, jatyadi taila, jatyadi ghrita, nirgundi taila, kaishora guggulu and *mahamanjisthadi kvatha.*

Nidranasha

Vyadhiharana rasayana, asvagandhadi churna, asvagandharista, kumudesvara rasa, brahmi vati, nidrodaya rasa and *nidrodaya vati.*

Nakhakotha

Vyadhiharana rasayana.

Netra Roga

Vyadhiharana rasayana, saptamrita lauha, triphala churna and *triphaladya ghrita.*

Netra Adhimansa

Chandrodaya varti.

Netradaha

Bhringarajasava, kamdudha rasa, chandrakala rasa, mukta pishti and *draksava.*

Nadikshinata

Gadamurari rasa, javaharmohra, vrihat kasturibhairava rasa and *vrihat vatachintamani rasa.*

Nadi Aniyamitata

Javaharmohra.

Nasura

Nirgundi taila, vatari rasa and *mahalakshmivilasa rasa.*

See *nadivrana.*

Nasa Roga

Rasa manikya and *sadbindu taila.*

Nasarsha

Nasarshohara taila.

Prameha

Somesvara rasa, mehamudgara rasa, tapyadi lauha, hemanatha rasa, chandrakala rasa, makardhvaja vati, shilajatvadi vati, sarivadi vati, medoharavidangadi lauha, devdarvyadyarista, vidangasava, pramehamihira taila, shrigopala taila, prameha-hara kvatha, svarnavanga, svarnabhupati rasa, chaturmukha rasa, pramehagajakeshari rasa, vrihat purnachandra rasa, pravalapanchamrita rasa, basantakusumakara rasa, vrihat vangesvara rasa, basantatilaka rasa, ratnagarbhapottali rasa, chandraprabha vati, ayaskriti, madhukasava, nishakatakadi kashaya, shukramatrika vati and *trivanga bhasma.*

Prameha Pidika

Madhusnuhi rasayana, kaishora guggulu, navayasa churna and *dhanvantara ghrita.*

Parsvashula

Soma yoga, puskaramula kalpa, sringa bhasma, hingvadi churna, svarnasamirapannaga rasa, kumudesvara rasa, draksharista, sitopaladi churna and *gadamurari rasa.*

Pandu

Kshayantaka rasa, shilajatvadi vati, parpati kalpa (*shothayukta pandu*), *manduraparpati, pranada parpati, agnimukha lauha, agnimukha mandura, tapyadi lauha, abhraka bhasma, ayaskriti, tara mandura, kasisa bhasma, lauha bhasma, lohasava, triphaladi lauha, punarnavadi mandura, panchamritlauha mandura, mandura vataka, dantyarista, drakshasava, parpatadyarista, manduradyarista, kamdeva ghrita, triphaladi kvatha svarnabhupati rasa, samirapannaga rasa, vyadhiharana rasayana, chaunsathaprahari pippala, agnisunu rasa, trimurti rasa, vrihat purnachandra rasa, muktapanchamrita rasa, navaratnarajamriganka rasa, nagarjunabhra rasa, pandupanchanana rasa, murchhantaka rasa* and *laghvananda rasa.*

Pipasa/Pitta Prakopa

Kharjuradi vati and *rasadi rasa.*

See *trishna* also.

Pravahika

Dugdha vati (*sangrahani*), *gangadhara churna, vrihat gangadhara churna, pravahikahara churna, dhanyapanchakarista, kutajarista, vatsakadi kashaya, mahagandhaka rasa, lavangabhraka bhasma* and *kutajaghana vati.*

Prasuti Roga

Maghabhra vati, saubhagya vati, saubhagyashunthi paka, dashmularista, mritasanjivani sura, dashmula kvatha, chaturmukha rasa and *pratapalankesvara rasa.*

Pliha Roga

Shilajatvadi vati, vijaya parpati, mandura parpati, vardhamana pippali rasayana, pranada parpati, jambira drava, asvinikumara rasa (with *indrayana svarasa*), *kravyada rasa, yakritaplihari lauha, rohitakarista, kumaryasava, pravalapanchamrita rasa* and *svarnabasantamalti rasa.*

Parinama Shula

Vijaya parpati, rasa sindura, avipattikara churna, shankha bhasma, sukumara ghrita, bhringarajasava, shulaharana yoga, dhatri lauha, dadimadi ghrita, shulagajakeshari rasa, muktashukti bhasma and *kapardika bhasma.*

Paktishula

Tara mandura and *triphaladi lauha.*

See *parinamashula* also.

Pradara

Pradarantaka lauha, pradarari lauha, pradaranashaka churna, pusyanuga churna, patrangasava, vasarista, ashoka ghrita, darvyadi kvatha, pradarantaka kvatha, pradarantaka rasa, pradararipu rasa, ashokarista, laghumalinibasanta rasa and *svarnabasantamalti rasa.*

Pama

Pamari lepa, kasisadi taila, somaraji taila, kaishora guggulu, panchanimbadi churna, mahamarichyadi taila and *mahamanjisthadi kvatha.*

Pakshaghata

Dhatura kshara, maharasnadi kvatha, asvagandharista, asvagandhadi churna, samirapannaga rasa, svarnasamirapannaga rasa, ekangavira rasa, khanjanikari rasa, chintamanichaturmukha rasa, vrihat vatachintamani rasa, vatakulantaka rasa, vatagajankusha rasa, rasaraja rasa, chaturbhuja rasa dashmula kvatha, yogendra rasa, karpasasthyadi taila, dhanvantara taila and *mahanarayana taila.*

Pidika

Sarivadi vati, sarivadyarista and *eladyarista.*

Palitya

Purnachandra rasa, bhrigaraja taila, amritabhallataka avaleha, nilibhrangyadi taila, bhrangamalaka taila and *anu taila.*

Pratishyaya/Pinasa

Dashmula kvatha, dashmula rasayana rasnadi churna, trikatu churna, naradiya lakshmivilasa rasa, gulabanaphsadi kvatha, gojihvadi kvatha, agnikumara rasa, amritakalanidhi rasa, asvinikumara rasa, tripurabhairava rasa, chandramrita rasa, chandrakanta rasa, tribhuvanakirti rasa and *panchavaktra rasa.*

Prasuta Jvara

Giloya satva, godanti bhasma, pratapalankesvara rasa, dashmularista, dashmula kvatha and *devadarvyadi kvatha.*

Pechisa

See *pravahika.*

Pittashayashotha

Tamra sindura, tamrachandrodaya, triphalasava and *trikatu churna.*

Pangu

Mahanarayana taila, prasarini taila, kshirabala taila, mahamasha taila, svarnabhupati rasa, samirapannaga rasa, mahavatavidhvansana rasa, vatagajankusha rasa and *maharasnadi kvatha.*

Pakvatisara

Agastisutaraja rasa.

Pralapa

Vrihat vatachintamani rasa, amarasundari vati, kalakuta rasa nasya, gadamurari rasa and *vatakulantaka rasa.*

Pitta Vikara

Kamdudha rasa, pittantaka rasa, rasadi rasa, sutashekhara rasa, chandrakala rasa and *pravala pishti.*

Paragarbhika

Sarvangasundara rasa.

Phuphaphusa Avarana Shotha

Panchasuta rasa.

Phiranga Roga

Malla sindura.

Phakka Roga

Balapanchabhadra rasa and *balajivana gutika.*

Bahumutrata

Tarkesvara rasa, vrihat purnachandra rasa, basantakusumakara rasa, bahumutrantaka rasa, vanga bhasma, trivanga bhasma, pramehantaka vati, pramehahara kvatha, vangesvara rasa and *shilajatvadi vati.*

Baddhakostha

Gandhaka rasayana and *manmatha rasa.*

See *kosthabaddhata* also.

Bandhyatva

Puspadhanva rasa, manmatha rasa and *phalaghrita.*

Bala Roga

Chandrashekhara rasa, balajvarankusha rasa, kumarakalyana rasa, kumarakalyana ghrita, balarogantaka rasa, balarka rasa, rasapipari, arvindasava, shankhapuspi taila, sarvangasundara rasa, arvindasava, dantodbhedagadantaka rasa, mukta bhasma, balajivana gutika, bala vati, muktadi vati and *balachaturbhadra churna.*

Badhirya

Badhiryanashaka taila, bilva taila, rasaraja rasa, tryodashanga guggulu, asvagandhadi churna and *asvagandharista.*

Bhagandara

Svarnabhupati rasa, chandrakanta rasa, vrihat purnachandra rasa, vatari rasa, mahalakshmivilasa rasa, ratnagarbhapottali rasa, mahamanjisthadi kvatha, rasa kapura, rasa, manikya, somesvara rasa, shilajatvadi vati, chirubilvadi kashaya, abhayarista, triphala guggulu, madhusnuhi rasayana, saptavinshati guggulu, vidangadyarista, avipattikara churna and *panchasakara churna.*

Bhrama

Eladi gutika, chintamanichaturmukha rasa, javaharmohra, basantakusumakara rasa, kamdudha rasa, gadamurari rasa, mahamriganka rasa, laghvananda rasa, sutshekhara rasa, asvagandhadi churna, brahmi vati and *asvagandharista.*

Mandagni

Yavaksharadi churna, yavanishadava churna, angurasava, madhvarista, tamra sindura, agnikumara rasa, agnisunu rasa, agnitundi vati, agnisandipana rasa, ajirnakantaka rasa, amritakalanidhi rasa, nagarjunabhra rasa, pashupata rasa, mandagnisanhara rasa, mahamriganka rasa, laghvananda rasa, gagan parpati and *agnimukha churna.*

Mutravarodha

Tila kshara, mulaka kshara, svarnabhupati rasa, chandrakanta rasa, somesvara rasa, kaharvan vati, sveta parpati, gokshuradi guggulu and *mutrakricchhantaka rasa.*

Mutrakricchha

Pipal kshara, mulaka kshara, ushirasava, dashmularista, devdarvyadyarista, kamdeva ghrita, trikantakadi kvatha, varunadi kashaya, asvinikumara rasa, panchatrinamula kvatha, chandrakala rasa, mutrakricchhantaka rasa, sarvatobhadra rasa, sutshekhara rasa, pranada gutika, brahatyadi kashaya, chandanasava, kaharvan vati, sveta parpati, gokshuradi guggulu, punarnavadi guggulu and *varunadi lauha.*

Mutraghata

Kshara kalpa, ushirasava, svarnabhupati rasa, chandrakanta rasa, kaharvan vati, sveta parpati and *gokshuradi guggulu.*

Manodosha

Manasamitra vataka, brahmi ghrita, brahmi vati, mukta pishti, akika pishti, rajata bhasma, asvagandharista, asvagandhadi churna, panchagavya ghrita, brahmi taila, kalyanaka ghrita chaturmukha rasa, chintamanichaturmukha rasa, vatakulantaka rasa, unmadagajakeshari rasa and *unmadagajankusha rasa.*

Mutra Vikara

Chandanasava, chittachandirasava, lodhrasava, kamdudha rasa, navaratnakalpamrita rasa, sarivadyasava, pravalapanchamrita rasa, varunashigru kashaya and *chandraprabha vati.*

Medovriddhi

Jambira drava, mahamanjisthadi kvatha, ardhangavatari rasa, trimurti rasa, vatagajankusha rasa, vatari rasa, medohara guggulu, navaka guggulu, vidangarista and *medohara vidangadi lauha.*

Madatya

Shrikhandasava, dhatryadi ghrita, rajata bhasma and *astanga lavana.*

Mastiska Vikara

Sarasvata churna, sarasvatarista, brahmi ghrita, brahmi vati, asvagandharista, asvagandhadi churna, chaitasa ghrita and *chaturmukha rasa.*

Mukha Roga

Irimedadi taila, khadiradi taila, jatyadi kvatha, khadiradi gutika, panchavalkala kvatha, rasa manikya and *karpuradi vati.*

Murchha

Ardhanarinatesvara rasa nasya, unmata rasa nasya, kamdudha rasa, gadamurari rasa, chaturbhuja rasa, vatakulantaka rasa, vatebhakeshari rasa, murchhantaka rasa and *sarvatobhadra rasa.*

Mutrashayashotha

Rasa sindura, chandanasava, ushirasava, chandraprabha vati, gokshuradi guggulu and *varunashigru kashaya.*

Mastiskavaranashotha

Panchasuta rasa and *dashmula kvatha.*

Mridu Asthi

Panchasuta rasa, lakshadi guggulu, abha guggulu, muktashukti bhasma, kukkutandatvaka bhasma and *kapardika bhasma.*

Mansarbuda

Tamra sindura and *dashmula kvatha.*

Mukhapaka

Irimedadi taila, vyadhiharana rasayana, kamdudha rasa, sutashekhara rasa, karpuradi vati and *khadiradi vati.*

Mutrasharkara

Sveta parpati, yava kshara, mulaka kshara, agastisutaraja rasa, punarnavadi guggulu, gokshuradi guggulu, trikantakadi kvatha, mutrakricchhantaka rasa and *varunashigru kashaya.*

Mukhadaurgandhya

Asvinikumara rasa, irimedadi taila, khadiradi vati and *karpuradi vati.*

Malavrodha

Arogyavardhini gutika, rechaka vati, sukhavirechana vati, sukhavirechana churna, triphala churna, panchasakara churna, tikshnavirechana churna, navajivana rasa, abhayarista and *avipattikara churna.*

Manovibhrama

Chandrodaya rasa, mansyadi kvatha, jatamansi churna phanta, asvagandhadi churna, asvagandharista, smritisagara rasa, sarasvatarista, sarasvata churna and *brahmi vati.*

Madhumeha

Chandrakanta rasa, pramehagajakeshari rasa, basantakusumakara rasa, vangesvara rasa, madhumehanashini gutika and *phalatrikadi kvatha.*

Mutratisara

Chandrakanta rasa and *vangesvara rasa.*

Mastiskaghata

Vatakulantaka ras, akika pishti, asvagandharista, brahmi vati, sarasvatarista, sarasvata churna and *javaharmohra.*

Mastiska Daurbalya

Brahmi ghrita, brahmi vati, srasvatarista, chaturbhuja rasa and *rajata bhasma.*

Manyastambha

Vatagajankusha rasa, singhanada guggulu, rasnadi guggulu and *maharasnadi kvatha.*

Yakrita Vikara

Panchasuta rasa, yakritaplihari lauha, kalameghasava, kumaryasava, rohitakarista, mandura parpati, manikya rasa, chavyakarista and *jambira drava.*

Yoshapasmara

Svarnasamirapannaga rasa.

See *apasmara.*

Yakrita Vriddhi

Yakritaplihari lauha, rohitakarista, kumaryasava, agnitundi vati and *asvakanchuki rasa.*

Yonishula/Yonidaha

Chandranshu rasa.

Yonibhransha

Changeryadi ghrita, mushakadi taila and *chandranshu rasa.*

Yonikandu

Chandranshu rasa.

Yakshma

Chaunsathaprahari pippala, sitopaladi churna, svarnabasantamalti rasa, yakshmari lauha and *drakshasava.*

Yoni Vikara

Basantakusumakara rasa and *pushyanuga churna.*

Raktapradara

Lodhrasava, ashokarista, vasa kvatha, pushyanuga churna, pradarantaka lauha, bolabaddha rasa, bola parpati, chandrakala rasa, chandrashekhara rasa, patrangasava trinakantamani pishti, pravala pishti, phalakalyanaka ghrita, shilajatvadi vati, gokshuradi churna, vatebhakeshari rasa, muktapanchamrita rasa and *raktapittakulakandana rasa.*

Rajayakshma

Abhraka bhasma, sringa bhasma, pravala chandraputi, svarnabasantamalti rasa, astangavaleha, chyavanaprasha avaleha, kumudesvara rasa, gadamurari rasa, chaturbhuja rasa, chandrakanta rasa, vijaya parpati, shilajatvadi lauha, yakshmantaka lauha, yakshmari lauha, panchamrita rasa, piyushasindhu rasa, mriganka rasa, mahamriganka rasa, balachandra rasa and *rajamriganka rasa.*

Romantika

Panchasuta rasa and *eladyarista.*

Rajorodha

Nastapuspantaka rasa and *rajahpravartini vati.*

See *kastartava/kastarajah* also.

Raktasrava/Raktapitta

Akika pishti, drakshadi kashaya, bhunimbadi kashaya, muktapanchamrita rasa, amritadi churna, shankara lauha, kravyada rasa, durvadi ghrita, kamdudha rasa, chandrakala rasa, chandrashekhara rasa, kaharvan vati, guduchyadi modaka, madhukadya gutika, shilajatvadi lauha, sarivadi vati, bola parpati, raktapittantaka lauha, gokshuradi churna, kanakasava, kamdeva ghrita, baladi ghrita, bolabaddha rasa, raktapittakulakandana rasa, sarvatobhadra rasa, sudhanidhi rasa, sutashekhara rasa, eladi vati and *nagakeshara churna.*

Raktarsha

Kamdudha rasa, kutajarista, bolabaddhu rasa, muktapanchamrita rasa, shankhodara rasa and *laghumalinibasanta rasa.*

Rakta Vikara

Kusthakalanala rasa, amritarnava lauha, guduchyadi lauha, kaishora guggulu, mahamanjusthadi kvatha, khadirarista, ekavinshati guggulu, saptavinshati guggulu, vyadhiharana rasayana, kanakarista, nimbadi churna, sarivadyasava, triphala ghrita, guduchyadi taila, chandanabalalakshadi taila and *chandanadi taila.*

Raktatisara

Gangadhara rasa, kutajarista, gokshuradi churna, nagakesharadi churna, bilvaphaladi churna, bhunimbadi churna, nrapativallabha rasa and *shankhodara rasa.*

See *raktapitta* also.

Rajodosha

Chandranshu rasa.

Raktachapa

Chintamani rasa, pravala chandraputi, mukta pishti, sarpagandha yoga and *yogendra rasa.*

Raktaprameha

Bolabaddha rasa, muktapanchamrita rasa and *gokshuradi churna.*

Raktavamana

Eladi vati, durvadi ghrita, vasa ghrita, vasavaleha, bolabaddha rasa and *raktapittakulakandana rasa.*

See *raktapitta* also.

Rasayana

Agastyaharitaki rasayana, chyavanaprasha avaleha, amritabhallataka avaleha, brahm rasayana, asvagandhadi avaleha, mushalipaka avaleha kusmanda rasayana, dhatri rasayana, makardhvaja rasayana and *navajivana rasa.*

Lasikarbuda

Svarnasamirapannaga rasa, tamra bhasma, vajra bhasma, vaikranta bhasma, shila sindura, kanchanara guggulu, dashmula kvatha and *nimbamritarista.*

Lasikagranthishotha

Nityananda rasa, slipadagajakeshari rasa and *shakhotaka kvatha.*

Vamana

Eladi churna, trikatu churna, tamra sindura, mayurapicchha bhasma, pippalavriksha tvaka bhasma, agastisutaraja rasa, sarvatobhadra rasa, eladi vati, chhardiripu vati, chhardiripu rasa, gadamurari rasa, nilakantha rasa and *vantihrada rasa.*

Visphota

Panchasuta rasa, rasa manikya, somesvara rasa, chandanabala lakshadi taila, jatyadi taila, haridrakhanda, kapardika bhasma, eladyarista, sarivadyasava, mahamanjisthadi kvatha, kaishora guggulu, panchatiktaghrita guggulu, saptavinshati guggulu and *chavyakarista.*

Vrana

Mahayogaraja guggulu, saptavinshati guggulu, kaishora guggulu, panchatiktaghrita guggulu, jatyadi ghrita, jatyadi taila, chopchinyadi churna, dashanga lepa, vranarakshasa taila, nirgundi taila, somraji taila, rasa manikya, sarivadyasava, khadirarista and *mahamanjisthadi kvatha.*

Vatarakta

Tala sindura, nimbadi churna, chavyakarista, mahamanjisthadyarista, mahamanjisthadi kvatha, kamdeva ghrita, rasa manikya, amritadi guggulu, kaishora guggulu, kusthakalanala rasa, nityananda rasa, vrihat purnachandra rasa, vatakulantaka rasa and *bolabaddha rasa.*

Vatanadishaithilya

Panchasuta rasa.

Vata Roga

Panchasuta rasa, svarnasamirapannaga rasa, svarnabhupati rasa, shuddha kuchla churna, dashmula kvatha, hargauri rasa, rasnadi guggulu, raktachandanadi churna, dashmularista, balarista, asvagandharista, dashmula taila, narayana taila, mahanarayana taila, mahamasha taila, lakshmivilasa taila, himsagara taila, maharasnadi kvatha, rasnasaptaka kvatha, bala asvagandhalakshadi taila, mahavatavidhvansana rasa, yogendra rasa, vishmustyadi vati, panchamritalauha guggulu, unmadagajakeshari rasa, trailokyachintamani rasa, navratnarajamriganka rasa, vrihat vatachintamani rasa, vatakulantaka rasa, vatagajankusha rasa, vatavidhvanshana rasa, vatari rasa, chintamanichaturmukha rasa, dashmula katutryadi kvatha, dhanvantara taila, ekangavira rasa, gandharvahastadi kashaya, karpasasthyadi taila and *prasarini taila.*

Visuchika

Tamra sindura, amritakalanidhi rasa, mrigamadasava, vrihat kasturibhairava rasa, basantatilaka rasa, grahnigajakeshari rasa, visuchividhvansana rasa, samiragajakeshari rasa and *sarvatobhadra rasa.*

Vatika Kasa

Tamra sindura, pravala bhasma, sitopaladi churna, chyavanaprasha avaleha, draksharista, samirapannaga rasa, pravala chandraputi, talishadi churna, vasavaleha and *vasarista.*

Vali

Purnachandrodaya rasa, asvakanchuki rasa, shankara lauha, rasayana and *vahikarana aushadhi.*

Viryakshinata

Asvagandhadi churna, kamdeva churna, narsingha churna, vidaryadi churna, madanaprakasha churna, shatavaryadi churna, narikelasava, kamdeva ghrita, shatavari ghrita, rasaraja rasa, shakravallabha rasa, kasturi vati, chandraprabha vati, shilajatvadi vati, kaminividravana rasa, puspadhanva rasa, phalaghrita, basantakusumakara rasa and *vangesvara rasa.*

Vajikarana

Makardhvaja rasayana, vanari gutika, mushalipaka avaleha, kaunchapaka avaleha, manmatha rasa, kamchudamani rasa and *asvagandhadi lehya.*

Vidradhi

Vidangarista, svarnabhupati rasa, dhanvantara ghrita, kaishora guggulu, gandharvahasta taila, misraka sneha, chopchinyadi churna, jambira drava, vidangasava, bolabaddha rasa, mahamriganka rasa, amavatari rasa, panchatiktaghrita guggulu and *mahamanjisthadi kvatha.*

Vrakkashotha

Vyadhiharana rasayana.

Vedana

Agastisutaraja rasa, vedanantaka rasa, vedanantaka churna, dashmula kvatha, guggulu kalpa, mahavatavidhvansana rasa, vatagajankusha rasa, maharasnadi kvatha, dashmula kvatha, asvagandhadi churna and *rasnasaptaka kashaya.*

Vatashula

Asvakanchuki rasa.

See *vata roga* also.

Visarpa

Dashanga lepa, rasa manikya, kaishora guggulu, sarivadyasava and *mahamanjisthadi kvatha.*

Vastishula

Hingvadi churna, varunadi kashaya, varunashigru kashaya, gokshuradi guggulu and *mutrakricchhantaka rasa.*

Vyanga

Lavangasava.

Vibandha

Abhayadi kvatha, aragvadhadi kashaya and *tarunyadi kvatha.*

See *kosthabaddhata* also.

Vicharchika

Sinduradi lepa, kasisadi ghrita, mahamarichyadi taila, rasamanikya and *rasottamadi lepa churna.*

Vipadika

Sarjarasa malhama, rasa manikya, and *sinduradi lepa.*

Virechana

Icchhabhedi rasa and *trivritta churna.*

Vatika Granthi

Kravyada rasa.

Vishama Jvara

Kalari rasa, chandrodaya rasa, nagarjunabhra rasa, mritasanjivani rasa, lakshminarayana rasa and *vishamajvarantaka lauha.*

Vyakulata

Gadamurari rasa.

Vismriti

Javaharmohra.

Visvachi

Pratapalankesvara rasa, tryodashanga guggulu, mahayograja guggulu, asvagandhadi churna, asvagandharista and *maha-rasnadi kvatha.*

Vidagdha Ajirna

Sarvatobhadra rasa.

Vatodara

Lashunadi vati, hinguvachadi churna and *tryodashanga guggulu.*

Sutika Roga

Sutikari rasa, sutikabharana rasa, vrihat sutikabharana rasa, vatakulantaka rasa, pratapalankesvara rasa, dashmula kvatha, dashmularista, mahagandhaka rasa, somesvara rasa and *somayoga.*

Soma Roga

Somnatha rasa, somesvara rasa, soma yoga and *basantakusu-makara rasa.*

Sangrahani

Hirnayagarbhapottali rasa, jatiphaladi vati, takra vati, jatiphaladi churna, dadimpaka vati, dugdha vati (sangrahani), parpati kalpa, dhanyapanchakarista, lai churna, karpurasava, kutajarista, rasa sindura, svarnasindura, agastisutaraja rasa, nrapativallabha rasa, pashupata rasa, piyushavalli rasa, piyushasindhu rasa, vrihat purnachandra rasa, vidyadharabhra rasa, mahagandhaka rasa, rambana rasa, lakshminarayana rasa, sindurabhushana rasa, agnikumara rasa, kanakasundara rasa, karpura rasa, grahanikapata rasa and *grahanigajakeshari rasa.*

See *grahani* also.

Sannipata

Hemagarbhapottali rasa, amritamanjari vati, sanchetana vati, saubhagya vati, rasa sindura, samirapannaga rasa, shivatandava rasa, sannipatabhairava rasa, ardhanarinatesvara rasa and *kalakuta rasa.*

Shirahshula

Amritadi taila, shirahshuladivajra rasa, rasnadi churna, navjivana rasa, kshayantaka rasa, amavatari vati, sirdardanashaka churna, pathyadi kvatha, madhukadi hima, vatebhakeshari rasa and *ardhanarinatesvara rasa* (*nasya*).

Stambhanahrasa

Anandada vati, jatiphaladi vati, purnachandrodaya rasa and *makardhvaja.*

Svarabheda

Eladi vati, khadiradi vati, kamdeva ghrita, madhukadya gutika, hingvadi churna and *mahamriganka rasa.*

Smritihrasa

Brahmi vati, sarasvata churna, rajatasindura, purnachandrodaya rasa, smritisagara rasa, basantakusumakara rasa, kamdudha rasa, rajata bhasma, sarasvatarista, brahmi ghrita, shankhapuspi panaka and *asvinikumara rasa.*

Svapnadosha

Chandrakala vati, chandanasava, chandraprabha vati, jatiphaladi vati, svarnavanga, vanga bhasma, trivanga bhasma, navratnakalpamrita rasa, purnachandra rasa, vrihat vangesvara rasa, agnitundi vati and *chandrakanta rasa.*

Snayushula

Mahayograja guggulu, svarnasindura, trailokyachintamani rasa, kaishora guggulu, dashmula kvatha and *maharasnadi kvatha.*

Sarvangashula

Chitrakadi churna, panchavaktra rasa, gadamurari rasa, dashmula kvatha, mahayograja guggulu, singhnada guggulu and *maharasnadi kvatha.*

Stri Roga

Ashokarista, sundari kalpa, phalaghrita, patrangasava, pradarantaka lauha and *pusyanuga churna.*

Sarvanga Roga

Navjivana rasa, asvagandharista, asvagandhadi churna, balarista and *kumaryasava.*

Sannipata Jvara

Mrigmadasava, mritsanjivani sura, samirapannaga rasa, panchavaktra rasa, naradiya lakshmivilasa rasa, kasturibhushana rasa and *amarasundari vati.*

Sandhishotha

Mahavishagarbha taila, vatavidhvansana rasa, gadamurari rasa, amira rasa, samirapannaga rasa and *dashmula kvatha.*

Stanya Dusti

Stanyashodhaka kashaya.

Sarvanga Shotha

Mandura kalpa, dashmula kvatha, punarnavadi guggulu, punarnavastaka kvatha, shothashardula taila, gokshuradi guggulu, jalodarari rasa, icchhabhedi rasa and *naracha rasa.*

Sthaulya

Shila sindura, mahalakshmivilasa rasa, kravyada rasa, vidangarista, medohara guggulu, navaka guggulu, tapyadi lauha, medohara vidangadi lauha and *trikatu churna.*

Sarvanga Vata

Mahayograja guggulu, samirapannaga rasa, mahavatavidhvansana rasa, balarista, maharasnadi kvatha, mahayograja guggulu, tryodashanga guggulu and *dashmula kvatha.*

Sujaka

Svarnavanga, anantamula kvatha, chandanasava, guduchi satva, pravala chandraputi, chopchinyadi churna, mrityunjaya rasa and *khanjanikari rasa.*

Shotha

Agastisutaraja rasa, dugdha vati (*shotha*), *punarnava churna, tapyadi lauha, agnimukha lauha, shothakalanala rasa, agnimukha mandura, tara mandura, shothari mandura, punarnavastaka kvatha* and *dashmula kvatha.*

Stabdhata

Basantatilaka rasa.

Sukha Roga

Balapanchabhadra rasa and *arvindasava.*

Suryavarta

Chandrakanta rasa, sutshekhara rasa, shirahshuladivajra rasa and *pathyadi kvatha.*

Sarvangadaha

Gadamurari rasa, chandanasava, ushirasava, chandrakala rasa, pravala chandraputi, mukta bhasma, chandanabala lakshadi taila, mukta pishti and *kamdudha rasa.*

Svedadhikya

Gadamurari rasa, kamdudha rasa, chandanasava, ushirasava, javaharmohra and *mukta bhasma.*

Sarvanga Kampa

Chaturbhuja rasa, kampavatari rasa, vanari gutika, asvagandhadi churna, asvagandharista, brahmi vati, sarasvatarista and *kaunchapaka avaleha.*

Stanyashosha

Chaunsathaprahari pippala.

Sanyasa

Malla sindura and *kalakuta rasa* (*nasya*).

Svitra

Ayaskriti, chitrakasava, gomurasava, avalgujadi lepa, madhusnuhi rasayana, kasisa bhasma, manibhadra guda, somraji or *bakuchi taila* and *bakuchi churna.*

Shula

Shulaharana yoga, shankha bhasma, avipattikara churna, hingavastaka churna, shulakuthara rasa, aditya gutika, amavatari vati, and *shivaksharapachana churna.*

Sveta Pradara

Pusyanuga churna, gokshuradi churna, ashokarista, pradarantaka lauha, patrangasava and *pradarantaka rasa.*

Shitapitta

Haridrakhanda, shitapittabhanjana rasa, khadirarista, sarivadyasava and *shirishadi kvatha.*

Svasa

Svasakuthara rasa, svasakasachintamani rasa, kanakasava, talisadi churna, chandrodaya rasa, chaunsathaprahari pippala, dashmula radayana, elakanadi kashaya, nayopanam kashaya and *vyaghri haritaki.*

See *tamaka svasa* also.

Hysteria

See *yoshapasmara.*

Malla sindura, chandranshu rasa, chandrodaya rasa, vrhat vatachintamani rasa and *vatakulantaka rasa.*

Hikka

Eladi gutika, tamra sindura, svarnamakshika bhasma, kachuradi churna, chaunsathaprahari pippala, vatebhakeshari rasa, mrigamadasava, mayurapicchha bhasma and *sutashekhara rasa.*

Hridaya Daurbalya

Arogyavardhini vati, kumudesvara rasa, chaturbhuja rasa, chintamanichaturmukha rasa, chaunsathaprahari pippala, javaharmohra, navratnakalpamrita rasa, arjunarista, basantakusumakara rasa and *yakuti rasayana.*

Halimaka

Kamalahara rasa, trimurti rasa, pandupanchanana rasa, murchhantaka rasa, muktapanchamrita rasa, patoladi kvatha, somesvara rasa, astangadashanga lauha, triphaladi kvatha/ phalatrikadi kvatha, parpatadyarista and *kamdeva ghrita.*

See *kamala* also.

Hridaya Shula

Nagarjunabhra rasa, gadamurari rasa, gulmakuthara rasa, chintamani rasa, vrihat purnachandra rasa, arjunarista, puskara guggulu and *hingvadi churna.*

Hridaya Roga

Hritkapata rasa, hritchintamani rasa, nagarjunabhra rasa, chintamani rasa, akika pishti, chandanasava, dhanvantara gutika, manikya bhasma, manikya pishti, mukta pishti, pravala pishti, arjunarista/parthadyarista, pravalapanchamrita rasa, hridyarnava rasa, jambira drava, kamaladi phanta, hemgarbhapottali rasa, prabhakara vati, hingukarpuradi vati and *vijaya parpati.*

Hritkshiprata

Hritchintamani rasa, javaharmohra and *chintamani rasa.*

Hanustambha

Vatagajankusha rasa, vidangasava and *dashmula kvatha.*

Hridavaranashotha

Mrityunjaya rasa.

Hridavarodha

Rasa manikya.

Hridadaha

Kamdeva ghrita.

Shighrapatana

Makardhvaja gutika, vanari gutika, kaminividravana rasa, kamchudamani rasa, mushalipaka avaleha, kaunchapaka avaleha, basantakusumakara rasa and *manmatha rasa.*

Shitanga Sannipata

Mrigamadasava, tala sindura, malla sindura, shila sindura, samirapannaga rasa, khanjanikari rasa and *chaturbhuja rasa.*

Slipada

Mahamanjisthadyarista, slipadagajakeshari rasa, nityananda rasa, mahalakshmivilasa rasa and *shakhotaka kvatha.*

Shiro Roga

Anu taila, svarnabhupati rasa, brahmi vati, shankhapuspi panaka, brahmi ghrita, asvagandhadi churna, asvagandharista, sarasvata churna and *sarasvatarista.*

Sharkara

Ashmarihara kashaya, varunadi kashaya and *varunashigru kvatha.*

Shopha

Loknatha rasa, mutrala kashaya, punarnavadi guggulu, gokshuradi guggulu, punarnavastaka kashaya, panchatrinamula kashaya and *gokshuradi kashaya.*

Shirah Kampa

Chaturbhuja rasa, vrihat vatachintamani rasa and *asvagandharista.*

See *kampavata* also.

Shitala

Panchasuta rasa.

Svasakricchhata

Malla sindura, samirapannaga rasa and *chaturbhuja rasa.*

See *svasa* also.

Shukrameha

Chandraprabha vati, chandanasava, svarnavanga, trivanga bhasma, vanga bhasma, pramehagajakeshari rasa, vrihat purnachandra rasa and *kamdhenu rasa.*

Shosha

Agnisunu rasa, panchamrita rasa, samiragajakeshari rasa, sitopaladi churna and *dhatupaustika churna.*

See *kshaya* also.

Shita Jvara

Asvinikumara rasa, shitabhanji rasa and *shitajvarari rasa.*

Svetakustha

Udayaditya rasa and *rasa manikya.*

See *svitra* also.

Shaktihrasa

Chaturbhuja rasa, navjivana rasa, shatavaryadi churna, dhatupaustika churna, vidaryadi churna and *balarista.*

Kshaya

Hemabhraka sindura, sitopaladi churna, hemgarbhapottali rasa, kshayantaka rasa, drakshasava, draksharista and *dashmularista.*

Kshatakshaya

Madhukadya gutika, sitopaladi churna and *kamdeva ghrita.*

Proprietary Medicine Index

Gastrointestinal System

Antacids

Acidiact tablet (Kottakal); 2 tablets tds or as required, Acidinol tablet (Ban); 2 tablets tds, Amalaki tablet (AIMIL); 2 tablets tds, Amlapittamishran suspension (Shri Dhootpapeshvar Limited); 1–2 teaspoonful (tsf) tds, Amlapittantak yog (Baidyanath); 2 tablets bid or as required, Himcocid suspension (Himalaya); 2 tsf tds, Nutral tablet (Nagarjuna); 1–2 tablets tds, Plantacid capsule/suspension (Solumiks); 1–2 capsule tds/2 tsf tds, Pittashekhara rasa (SDL); 1–2 tablets od/bid.

Carminative and Digestants

D2D tablet (Alarsin); 1–2 tablets to be chewed slowly before or after meal, Dilapsin tablet/syrup (Solumiks); 2 tablets bid or as required/2 tsf tds, Gason syrup (Nagarjuna); 2–3 tsf tds, Gaisantaka vati (Baidyanath); 2 tablets bid, Gastrex tablet (Ban); 2 tablets tds, Ojus syrup/tablet (Charak); 1–2 tsf tds/ 1–2 tablets bid to be chewed, Pep-up syrup/tablet (Vasu); 2 tsf tds/1–2 tablets tds, Colicarmin syrup (Ban); 2 tsf bid to tds.

Antidiarrheal

Bactefar syrup (Ayulabs); 1–2 tsf tds, Berbenterone tablet (Sandu); 2 tablets tds, Diarex tablet (Himalaya); 1–2 tablets bid, Dysentrol tablet (Dhanvantari); 1–2 tablet tds, Entostal tablet (Solumiks); 2 tablets tds.

Antiemetic

Vomiteb tablet/syrup (Charak); 1 tab. to be chewed as required/2 tsf tds (***Note:*** Contraindicated in meningitis, uremia, acute abdomen), Emilet capsule (Salveo); 1–2 capsule bid to tds.

Hepatobiliary Preparation

Amlycure DS capsule/syrup (Aimil); 2 capsule tds/2 tsf tds, Cytozen capsule/syrup (Charak); 1 capsule bid/2 tsf tds, Jaundex syrup (Sandu); 2 tsf tds, Liv 52 DS syrup/ tablet (Himalaya); 1–2 tsf/tablets bid, Livex capsule/syrup (Ban); 1 capsule/1–2 tsf tds, Livomyn tablet/syrup (Charak); 2 tablets/2 tsf tds, Nirocil tablet/syrup (Solumiks); 1 tablet/ 2 tsf tds; Stimuliv tablet (Francoindian); 2 tablets tds, Vasuliv syrup (Vasu); 2 tsf tds, Vimliv tablet/syrup (Solumiks); 2 tablets/tsf tds.

Laxatives

Golax powder (Francoindian); 2 tsf at bedtime, Herbolax capsule/tablet (Himalaya); 2–3 capsule/tablet or as required at bedtime (Contraindicated in intestinal obstruction and pregnancy), Isova powder (Vasu); 1–2 tsf at bedtime, Nityam churna (Zandu); ½–1 tsf or as required at bedtime, Myrilax tablet (SDL); 1 tablet at bedtime, Picrolax capsule (Himalaya); 2 capsule at bedtime, Regulax tablet (Charak); 1 tablet at bedtime.

Anorectal Preparation

Amroid capsule/ointment (Aimil); 2 capsules tds/to be applied topically, Arshonyt tablet/ointment (Charak); 2 tablets bid/to be applied topically, Arsh hita tablet/ointment (SDL); 2–3 tablets tds/to be applied topically, Arshol capsule (Ban); 1 capsule tds, Kultab tablet (Vasu); 1–2 tablets tds, Pilex tablet/ointment (Himalaya); 2 tablets bid/to be applied topically, Pilocid tablet/ointment (Kottakkal); 2 tablets tds/to be applied topically.

Ulcer Healing Formulations

Alsarex tablet (Charak); 2 tablets bid to tds, Protekt tablet (Nagarjuna); 1–2 tablets bid to tds, Zulcer capsule (Gufic); 2 capsules bid.

Appetizers and Antispasmodics

Aptizoom syrup (Charak); 2–3 tsf tds, Trikatu syrup (Himalaya); 1 tsf tds, Zanduzyme tablet (Zandu); 1 tablet bid, Ojus syrup (Charak); 2 tsf tds, Himcospaz soft capsule (Himalaya); 2 capsule stat. followed by 1 capsule 8 hourly (Contraindicated in pregnancy), Colicarmin syrup (Ban); 2 tsf tds.

Cardiovascular System

Antianginal Preparation

Abana tablet (Himalaya); 2 tablets bid, Arjin tablet (Alarsin); 2 tablets tds to qid, Favordil capsule (UAP); 1–2 capsule bid, Prabhakara mishran tablet (Dhanvantari); 1 tablet bid.

Antihypertensives

Digit capsule (Vasu); 1 capsule bid to tds, Sarpgandha mishran tablet (Dhanvantari); 1–2 tablets tds, Siledin tablet (Alarsin); 1 tablet bid, Serpina tablet (Himalaya); 1 tablet bid, Cardostab tablet (Nagarjuna); 1 tablet bid.

Cardiotonic Preparation

Arjunin capsule (Charak); 2 capsules tds to qid, Hridroga chintamani rasa (SDL); 1 tablet od or bid, Marmotone tablet (Manil); 2 tablets bid.

Hemostatic Preparation

Ayapon tablet (Alarsin); 2 tablets bid to tds, Point capsule (Ayulabs); 1–2 capsule bid, Posex forte capsule (Charak); 2 capsules tds, Raktastambhaka tablet (SDL); 1 tablet bid, Styplon tablet (Himalaya); 1–2 tablets bid.

Respiratory System

Anti-asthmatic Preparation

Bresol tablet/syrup (Himalaya); 2 tablets/tsf tds, Ephenin tablet (Sandu); 1–2 tablets tds, Fizzle capsule (Ayulabs); 1–2 capsule bid to tds, Respikot tablet (Kottakkal); 1 tablet tds, Svaskalp tablet (Dabur); 1–2 tablets bid, Spasma syrup (Charak); 2–3 tsf tds.

Antitussive Preparation

Crux syrup (Ban); 1–2 tsf tds, Dekofcyn syrup (Alarsin); 2 tsf tds, Honicof syrup (Solumiks); 2 tsf tds, Jufex forte syrup (Aimil); 2 tsf tds, Koflet syrup (Himalaya); 2 tsf tds, Kuka syrup (Multani); 2 tsf tds, Mincof syrup (SDL); 2 tsf tds, Zeal syrup (Vasu); 2 tsf tds.

Aromatic Inhalations

Halin soft capsule (Nagarjuna); to be inhaled with vapours, Maha inhaler (Amrutanjana) for inhalation.

Central Nervous System

Analgesics and Antipyretics

A-flu-o-cil tablet (SDL); 1–2 tablets tds, Feverex syrup (Dhanvantari); 2–3 tsf tds, Godanti mishran tablet (Dhanvantari); 1–2 tablets tds, Mahasudarshan ghanvati (Baidyanath); 2 tablets tds, Plugit capsule (Vasu); 1–2 capsule bid to tds, Tribhuvan mishran tablet (Dhanvantari); 2–3 tablets tds, Trishun tablet (Zandu); 1 tablet daily.

Antidepressants and Anxiolytics

Alert capsule (Vasu); 1–2 capsule bid, Siotone capsule (Albert david); 1 capsule bid, Nervomine tablet (Francoindian); 1–2 tablets tds, Stressan tablet (Sandu); 1 tablet bid, Sobex capsule (Ayukalp); 1 capsule tds, Memtone syrup (Aimil); 2 tsf tds.

Memory Boosters

Brahmi capsule (Kottakkal); 2 capsules bid, Brento syrup (Zandu); 2 tsf bid or as required, Cognium syrup (Charak); 2 tsf bid, Dimag doshahari tablet (Baidyanath); 2 tablets bid, Mentat syrup (Himalaya); 2 tsf tds, Smriti granules (Nagarjuna); 1 tsf bid.

Sedatives and Tranquilizers

Bravobol capsule (Ban); 2 capsule at bedtime, Stresscom capsule (Dabur); 1–2 capsule bid, Stresswin capsule (Baidyanath); 1 capsule bid.

Infections

Immunity Boosters

Extrammune tablet (Charak); 1 tablet bid, Septilin syrup/tablet (Himalaya); 2 tsf tds/2 tablets bid, Step capsule (Vasu); 1–2 capsules bid to tds.

Medicines for Malaria

Chirakin tablet (Zandu); 2 tablets tds (Contraindicated in pregnancy), MP6 capsule (Vasu); 1 capsule tds followed by bid, Malaria mixture syrup (UAP); 1–4 tds bid to tds.

Medicines for Protozoal and Viral Infection

Amoebica tablet (Baidyanath); 2 tablets tds, Bactefar capsule (Ayulabs); 2 capsules tds, Virocil capsule/syrup (Arar); 2 capsules tds/2 tsf tds.

Anthelminthics

Cruminil syrup (Charak); Adult: 2–3 tsf tds, Children: Half of the adult dose, Krimihar syrup (Dhanvantari); 3–4 tsf tds, children: half of the adult dose.

Endocrine System

Medicines for Diabetes

Amree plus capsule (Aimil); 1–2 tablet bid before meal, Asphal capsule (Nagarjuna); 1 capsule bid, Diabac tablet (Bacfo); 1–2 tablet bid, Diabecon tablet (Himalaya); 2 tablets bid, Diarid capsule (Nagarjuna); 2 capsules tds, Glucova tablet (Vasu); 1–2 tablet bid to tds, Glycoban capsule (Ban); 1–2 capsule half an hour before meal, Madhumeha kusumakara rasa (SDL); 1–2 tablet od to bid, Zepter tablet (Solumiks); 2 tablets bid before meal.

Fertility Enhancers

Afrodet plus capsule (Solumiks); 1 capsule bid, Count plus granules (Nagarjuna); 2 tsf bid, Fortege capsule (Alarsin); 1–2 tablets bid to tds, Speman tablet (Himalaya); 2 tablets bid, Vysex dragee (Ban); 1 dragee bid.

Sex Stimulants

Vanari kalp granules (Sandu); 1 tsf tds, Afrol plus capsule (Solumiks); 2 capsule od at bedtime, Confido tablet (Himalaya); 1 tablet bid, Himcolin gel (Himalaya); Topical application (as directed), Makaradhvaj rasayan tablet (Ayukalp); 1 tablet bid, Semento capsule (Aimil); 1–2 capsule tds.

Medicines for Thyroid Dysfunction

Gaytarin tablet (Arya aushadhi); 1–2 tablet bid to tds, Metostab tablet (Yamuna); 1 tablet bid, Reguthyro (Biosurge); 1 tablet bid.

Gynecological Disorders

Falaa gold capsule (Ban); After confirmation of pregnancy, 2 capsules early in the morning empty stomach for 10 days (do not eat meal up to 2 hours of taking medicine), Gestone syrup (Zandu); 2–3 tsf tds, Femiplex tablet (Charak); 2 tablets bid in poor lactations, Galacol tablet (Charak); 2 tablets tds in poor lactations, Leptaden tablet (Alarsin); 2 tablets tds after delivery, Maa-lact granules (Solumiks); 1–2 tsf bid, Shataverex granules (Zandu); 1–2 tsf tds with milk.

Genitourinary System

Urinary Antiseptics

Alka 5 syrup (Charak); 2–3 tsf tds, Bangshil tablet (Alarsin); 2 tablets bid to tds, Renalka syrup (Himalaya); 2 tsf tds, Shitprabha tablet (SDL); 1–2 tablets bid.

Vulvovaginal Conditions

Leucorid tablet (Nagarjuna); 1 tablet bid, Lucogyl capsule (Ban); 1 capsule tds, Lumital tablet (Solumiks); 2 tablets tds, Myron tablet (Alarsin); 2 tablets bid to tds, V-gel (Himalaya); for topical application.

Menstrual Irregularities

Amycordial syrup/capsule (Aimil); 2 tsf/capsules tds for 3 months, Ashotone syrup/tablet (Solumiks); 1–2 tsf/1 tablet tds for 3 consecutive cycles, Evecare syrup/capsule (Himalaya); 2–3 tsf/1 capsule tds, Femiforte tablet (Charak); 2 tablets tds, M2-tone syrup (Charak); 3 tsf tds, Menocramp tablet (Solumiks); 1 tablet tds, Menoril forte capsule (Ban); 2 capsules tds, Meryton syrup (Vasu); 2–3 tsf tds, Normen tablet (Nagarjuna); 2 tablets bid, Ovarin capsule (Ban); 1 capsule tds, Senovila tablet (Solumiks); 2 tablets bid.

Menopausal Syndrome

Evanova capsule (Charak); 1 capsule bid, Menosan tablet (Himalaya); 1 tablet bid.

Uterine Sedatives

Amystop-G capsule (Aimil); 2 capsules tds, Ashoka compound (Sandu); 4 tsf bid, Ashotone syrup (Solumiks); 2 tsf tds, Femitone syrup (Nagarjuna); 2 tsf tds.

Benign Prostatic Hypertrophy

Himplasia tablet (Himalaya); 1 tablet bid, Prosteez tablet (Charak); 2 tablets bid, Ural-BPH capsule (Vasu); 1 capsule bid.

Renal Calculi

Calcurosin capsule/syrup (Ban); 1–2 capsule/tsf tds, Cristone capsule (Ayulabs); 1 capsule bid to tds, Cystone tablet/syrup (Himalaya); 2 tablets/tsf tds, Neeri tablet/syrup (Aimil); 2 tablets/2–3 tsf tds, Ural capsule/syrup (Vasu); 1 capsule/1–2 tsf bid to tds.

Diuretics

Aluretic tablet (Alarsin); 1–2 tablet bid to tds (Last dose not to be given late in the evening), Urexynol tablet (Ban); 2 tablets bid to tds.

Nutrition

Hematopoietics

Amyron tablet/syrup (Aimil); 1 tablet/2 tsf bid, Abhraloha tablet (SDL); 1–2 tablet bid, Blossom capsule (Ayulabs); 1–2 capsule bid, Efiplus capsule (Solumiks); 1 capsule bid, Feroliv forte capsule (Ban); 1 capsule bid, Haematab tablet (Nagarjuna); 1 tablet bid, Manoll capsule (Charak); 1 capsule bid, Manoll syrup (Charak); 2 tsf tds.

Tonics

Alpitone syrup (Zandu); 1 tsf bid, Cheerup syrup (Ayulabs); 2 tsf tds, Fasto powder (Adfac labs); 1–2 tsf bid, Viton 99 syrup (Ban); 2 tsf tds, Spiruwin active tablet (Baidyanath); 1–2 tablets bid, Swamla compound (SDL); 2 tsf bid, Vigoroll syrup (Charak); 1 tsf bid.

Immunomodulators

Cruel AT tablet (Ayukalp); 1 tablet bid, Immumod tablet (Wockardt); 1 tablet bid, Immuno plus granules (Nagarjuna); 1 tsf bid, Oxitard capsule (Himalaya); 1–2 capsule bid.

Anti-obesity

Defet-5 capsule (Ayulabs); 1–2 capsule tds, Simlim tablet (Vasu); 1 tablet bid, Ayurslim tablet (Himalaya); 1 tablet bid, Lipan capsule (Ban); 1 capsule tds, Liporid tablet (Nagarjuna); 1 tablet bid, Obenyl (Charak); 2 tablets tds.

Musculoskeletal System

Antirheumatics

Arthrella tablet (Charak); 1 tablet tds, Astavargakashayam tablet (Kottakkal); 2–3 tablets bid, Dazzle capsule (Vasu); 1 capsule bid to tds, Myostal forte tablet (Solumiks); 1 tablet bid to tds, Muscalt forte tablet (Aimil); 1 tablet tds, Penwel capsule (Ayulabs); 1 capsule tds, R.compound tablet (Alarsin); 2 tablets tds, R.pairyn tablet (Ban); 2 tablets tds, Rasrajeshvara rasa (SDL); 1 tablet od to bid, Rheumarid tablet (Nagarjuna); 1 tablet bid, Rheumat 90 liquid (Nagarjuna); 2–3 tsf tds, Rhue capsule (Ban); 1–2 capsule bid, Rhukot tablet (Kottakkal); 2 tablets tds, Rumalaya forte tablet (Himalaya); 1 tablet bid.

Gout

G-amrita capsule (SDH); 2 capsules tds, Arthosurg-G tablet (Biosurge); 1 tablet tds.

Neuromuscular Formulations

Neuron capsule (Prakruti); 1 capsule tds, Rhue gold capsule (Ban); 1 capsule bid, Rhumo gold capsule (Dhanvantari); 1 capsule bid.

Painkillers

Shallaki tablet (Vasu); 1 tablet bid, Sallaki plus tablet (Gufic); 1 tablet bid, Sallaki -XT tablet (Gufic); 1 tablet bid, Sallaki MR tablet (Gufic); 1 tablet bid, Sallaki forte tablet (Gufic); 1 tablet bid, Sallaki 600 tablet (Gufic); 1 tablet bid.

Rubefacient

Dazzle oil/oint/cool cream (Vasu); to be applied topically, Mobyl oil (Ayulabs); to be applied topically, Myostal liniment/gel (Solumiks); to be applied topically, Pyroflex liniment/gel (Solumiks); to be applied topically, Rheumat liniment (Nagarjuna); to be applied topically, Rhue oil (Ban); to be applied topically, Rhukot gel (Kottakkal); to be applied topically, Rumalaya liniment/gel (Himalaya); to be applied topically.

Calcium Supplements

Bon fit capsule (Ayulabs); 1 capsule bid, Bonton capsule/active granules/DQ tablet (Vasu); 1 capsule bid/2 tsf bid/1 tablet od, Gandha tailam capsule (Kottakkal); 1–2 capsule bid, Myostal SB tablet (Solumiks); 1 tablet bid, Calciost tablet (Ayukalp); 1 tablet bid, Reosto tablet (Himalaya); 1 tablet bid, Bonheal syrup (Aimil); 1–2 tsf bid.

Eye, ENT and dental

Eye Formulations

Fineye eye drops (Nagarjuna); to be applied in the eyes, Isotine eye drops (Jagat pharma); to be applied in the eyes, Netrol eye drops (Dhanvantari); to be applied in the eyes, Ophthacare eye drops (Himalaya); to be applied in the eyes.

Nose and Throat Conditions

Bresol-NS drops (Himalaya); to be instilled in each nostril, Cephagraine tablet/nasal drops (Charak); 2 tablets tds/to be instilled in each nostril, Migrakot tablet (Kottakal); 2 tablets tds.

Ear Conditions

Kanol ear drops (Dhanvantari); 2–3 drops 3–4 times a day, Karnabindu ear drops (UAP); 2–4 drops 2–3 times a day.

Dental Conditions

G-32 tablet (Alarsin); to be applied over the teeth and gums, Gum-tone powder/paste (Charak); to be used as tooth powder/toothpaste, Trudent toothpaste (Ban).

Skin

Antiallergics

Alleryn tablet (Ban); 1-2 tablets tds, Allergin granules (Nagarjuna); 1 tsf bid, Cutis oil/dusting powder/capsule (Vasu); to be applied topically/1-2 capsule bid, Dermafex oil/cream (Ban); to be applied topically, Urtiplex capsule/lotion (Charak); 1 capsule bid/to be applied topically, Histablock tablet (JRK); 1 tablet bid.

Skin Conditions

Purin capsule (Ayukalp); 1-2 capsules tds, Radona tablet/syrup (Solumiks); 2 tablets tds/2 tsf tds, Purodil syrup/ointment (Aimil); 2 tsf tds/to be applied typically, Dermafex capsule (Ban); 1 capsule tds, Lippu oil/ointment (JRK); to be applied topically,

Psoriasis

777 oil (JRK); to be applied topically, Psorolin ointment/oil (JRK); to be applied topically, Imupsora ointment (Charak); to be applied topically, Imupsora tablet (Charak); 2 tablets bid, Pesin tablet (JRK); 1 tablet bid, Psorakot tablet/gel (Kottakkal); 2 tablet tds/to be applied topically, Psoria oil (Nagarjuna); to be applied topically.

Acne

Acnovin ointment/capsule (Vasu); to be applied topically/1 capsule tds, Clarina ointment (Himalaya); to be applied topically, Pimplex cream (Unexo); to be applied topically, Purim tablet (Himalaya); 1-2 tablet bid, Skinelle cream (Charak); to be applied topically.

Pigmentation Disorders

Caratole E tablet (JRK); 1 tablet bid, Melatru ointment (Salveo); to be applied topically, Pigmento tablet/ointment (Charak); 2 tablets bid to tds,/to be applied topically, Tolenorm oil/ ointment (JRK); to be applied topically.

Hair and Scalp Preparation

Anagen grow serum (JRK); to be applied topically, Dano oil (JRK); to be applied topically, Hairzone solution (Himalaya); to be applied topically, Sesa capsule/oil/Shampoo (Ban); 1 capsule bid to tds/to be applied topically, Suvarna hair Vitalizer/ shampoo (Ban); to be applied topically, Trichup capsule/oil (Vasu); 1 capsule tds/to be applied topically.

Wound and Scars

Cutfar ointment (Ban); to be applied topically, Miniscar cream (Charak); to be applied topically, WH5 ointment (Gufic); to be applied topically.

Antifungals

Dadhar oint (Dhanvantari); to be applied topically, Six-C ointment (Ban); to be applied topically, Cutis ointment/dusting powder (Vasu); to be applied topically.

Bathing Soaps and Sanitizers

Aactaril soap (Himalaya), Dermafex soap (Ban), Nagarjuna bath soap (Nagarjuna), Purehands gel (Himalaya), Psorolin soap (JRK).

Other Formulations

Pediatrics

Ban baby oil/soap (Ban), Balkadu syrup (Sandu); 5–10 drops according to the age thrice a day, Berbenterone pediatric syrup (Sandu); Infant: 1 mL tds-qid, Children (1–2 years): 2 mL tds-qid, Children (2–4 years): 4 mL tds-qid, Bonnisan drops/ liquid (Himalaya); Drops: Infants up to 1 month: 5–10 drops tds, 1 month–6 months: 10–20 drops tds/Liquid: Infants up to 1 month: ½ tsf tds, 1 month–6 months: 1 tsf tds, 6 months–3 years: 2 tsf tds, Bonnispaz drops (Himalaya); 4 drops initially followed by 2 drops bid to tds, Caspa drops (Vasu); Infants up to 6 months: 5–10 drops tds 15 minutes before feeding, 6 months–2 years: 10–20 drops, Colicarmin drops (Ban); Infants 6 months–1 year: 3–5 drops tds to qid, Children 1–3 years: 4–6 drops tds, Livomyn drops (Charak); 10–20 drops tds to qid, Paedritone drops/syrup (Charak); Drops: Infants up to 1 month: 8–10 drops, 1 month–6 months: 15–20 drops, 6 months–1 year: ½–1 tsf tds to qid/1–5 years: 2 tsf tds, above 5 years: 3 tsf tds.

Geriatrics

Banovit tablet (Ban); 2 tablets tds, Geriforte tablet/syrup (Himalaya); 1–2 tablets bid/1–2 tsf bid, Kayamrit tablet (Ayukalp); 1 tablet bid, Shilajit capsule (Dabur); 2 capsules bid, Stresscom capsule (Dabur); 1 capsule bid.

Bibliography

1. Acharya Siddhinandan Mishra. Rasratnasamucchya, Chaukhambha Orientalia, Varanasi.
2. Ayurved Sar Sangrah, Shri Baidyanath Ayurved Bhavan Ltd, Naini (Prayagraj).
3. Chintamani, K Rama Chandra Reddy, Chaukhambha Orientalia, Varanasi.
4. G Prabhakara Rao. Cakradatta, Chaukhaba Orientalia, Varanasi.
5. Gururaj Sharma Mishra. Ayurved Prakash, Chaukhamba Bharti Academy, Varanasi.
6. Kaviraj Atridev Gupta. Ashtanga Hridayam, Chaukhambha Prakashan, Varanasi.
7. KR Srikantha Murthy. Sharngdhar Sanhita, Chaukhambha Orientalia, Varanasi.
8. Pt Kashinath Shastri. Rastarangini, Motilal Banarasidas, Mumbai.
9. Pt Kashinath Shastri and Gorakhnath Chaturvedi. Charak Sanhita, Chaukhambha Bharti Academy, Varanasi.
10. Pt Ram Raksha Pathak. Therapeutic guide to Ayurvedic Medicine, Shri Baidyanath Ayurved Bhawan Pvt Ltd, New Delhi.
11. Raghuvir Prasad Trivedi. Rashtriya Chikitsa Siddha Yoga Samgraha, Chaukhamba Sanskrit Series Office, Varanasi.
12. Ramnivas Sharma and Surendra Sharma. Vaidyachintamani, Chaukhamba Sanskrit Pratishthan, New Delhi.

13. Raskamdhenu, Chaukhambha Orientalia, Varanasi.
14. Satyendra Mishra. Bhavprakash, Chaukhamba Surbharti Prakashan, Varanasi.
15. Shrilakshmipati Shastri. Yogratnakar, Chaukhambha Prakashan, Varanasi.
16. Siddhinandan Mishra. Raspaddhati, Chaukhambha Orientalia, Varanasi.
17. Yadavji Trikamji Acharya. Siddha Yoga Sangraha, Shri Baidyanath Ayurved Bhavan Ltd, Naini (Prayagraj).

Index

A

B

C

D

G

H

J

K

L

U

V

Y